Practical Iridology

Using the Eye as a Guide to Health Risks and Wellbeing

Revised & Expanded Edition

Peter Jackson-Main

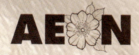

AE N

Figure 1.1, courtesy of Danny Woodmansey
Figures 1.2, 2.1, 2.4, 2.6, 2.13 courtesy of Andrew Mason

First published in 2023 by
Aeon Books Ltd

British Library Cataloguing in Publication Data

A C.I.P. for this book is available from the British Library

ISBN: 978–1–80152–115–4

Printed in Great Britain

www.aeonbooks.co.uk

CONTENTS

This volume is dedicated to my dear friends Angela and Peter Bradbury, founder members of the Guild of Naturopathic Iridologists and leading lights of the iridology community in the United Kingdom. Both have now passed on, but, while here, they were among my closest allies in everything that I did for iridology. Angela, a brilliant teacher and practitioner of iridology, whose encyclopedic knowledge will be much missed, passed a few days before I wrote this: I know she would have been delighted to know that this new edition of my book was on its way.

Endless love and thanks is also due to my wife, Anji, for her enduring support and belief in me, and for her own inspired teaching and practice in iridology. Her strongly worded encouragement for me to approach a publisher again after nearly 20 years provided the initial thrust that powered this to completion.

Huge thanks and respect also to my teachers, most notably Dr. Richard Schulze, who was my biggest inspiration in the early days, and whose friendship and support I continue to benefit from.

I am indebted to the College of Naturopathic Medicine (CNM), and particularly to its Principal, Hermann Keppler, for the opportunities, over the last 20 years of teaching there, to develop and refine my approach in the one place where it is always going to get the most exacting scrutiny: the classroom. CNM has taken me to the heart of its project to spread the knowledge of naturopathy and Natural Medicine as far and as wide as possible around the world and has been a beacon of the incandescent common sense of Natural Medicine in a world

Lastly, my thanks to Andrew Mason and Danny Woodmansey for additional graphics and images—Andrew in particular, as he was also responsible for the excellent 2019 update of my own iris chart.

To call **Peter Jackson-Main** my student would be an understate-
ment, because from the moment I first met him, I recognized
his ability, his wisdom, his knowledge, and his willingness to learn.
In fact, he reminded me . . . of me!

I was a student of the late Dr. Bernard Jensen, the man responsible for the research, further study, and advancement of iridology
in the last century. He authored his now classic work, *Iridology: The
Science and Practice in the Healing Arts*, in the 1950s, when I was born.
Beyond an iridologist, he also was a great natural doctor, herbalist, and chiropractor, operating his famous Hidden Valley Health
Ranch in Escondido, California, where I trained and apprenticed
with him. I was also a student of the late Dr. John Raymond Christopher, who was America's greatest herbalist in the last century,
and also an iridologist and a friend of Dr. Jensen. I trained and
interned with Dr. Christopher and taught side by side with him,
and he allowed me to be the head instructor of his famous School
of Natural Healing in Utah. You could say that I was groomed in
a Golden Age of iridology, herbology, and natural healing between
the two giants in the field in the twentieth century.

Dr. Christopher was asked to teach a course in herbal medicine
in Cambridge, UK, but he did not feel up to making this international journey, so he asked if I would teach as his replacement.
That is when I first met Peter, over 40 years ago, in Cambridge.
From the moment I met him it was obvious that I had a colleague,
someone like me who would carry on the work of my great teachers,
and also the work I had been doing in my own clinic for decades.

Peter's work on iridology is just the way I like it, and also the
way my famous teachers before me liked it: Commonsense, Simple,

Richard Schulze operated his now famous Natural Healing Clinic in
Hollywood and Malibu, California, and has been the owner of Dr. Schulze's
Herbal Products Company for the last 50 years.

and Practical. After all, what good is any clinical tool if the end result isn't the patient learning more about themselves, so they can adjust their lifestyle to get more quality and quantity out of life. Isn't that the bottom line? Quality and quantity! To feel great so you have the health and energy to do all the things you want to do in life, and to be able to do that for as long as possible.

Medicine today is far too complex—often the patient gets left behind in the dark. Doctors don't tell their patients much, figuring they don't understand anatomy, physiology, biochemistry, immunology, whatever. Peter's work, unlike conventional medicine, is to help the patient learn more about themselves, so they can fine-tune their lifestyle and make better choices, to get the most out of life. What is better than gaining further knowledge about yourself, so you make the right lifestyle choices? If that's not winning the game, I don't know what is.

In 1997, during an iridology conference in California, I had the pleasure of meeting Peter Jackson-Main for the first time. Our shared attendance at this event, where we eagerly anticipated Dr. Daniele Lo Rito's presentation on new theories, provided us with a profound insight into the multiple layers that can be revealed through an iris assessment.

It is with great honour that I write this foreword for Peter's remarkable book. Through his extensive experience, as both an iridology practitioner and a gifted teacher, Peter has skilfully reorganized the teachings of past masters into a contemporary framework, incorporating his own terminology. His eloquent writing style captivates readers, guiding them through the intricate world of constitutional elements. With thoughtful diagnostic questions and practical recommendations, Peter strives to establish a state of balance and harmony within individuals, known as homeostasis.

In his book, Peter emphasizes that iridology holds something of value for everyone interested in unravelling the underlying dynamics of health and disease. He eloquently explains that once we grasp the true essence of the iris, it can serve as a profound insight into both the inner reality of a person and the external manifestation of bodily ailments.

Peter and I share a common belief in the significance of focusing on the positive aspects when engaging with iridology. We wholeheartedly agree that this practice is not solely about what information the iris reveals, but, rather, about the actions and choices one makes based on that knowledge.

In summary, Peter Jackson-Main's book represents a milestone in the field of iridology. It is a testament to his dedication,

---

Toni Miller, ND, DHM, MII, CCII, Fellow Ir., is a leading Australian iridology teacher, researcher, and lecturer. She has been teaching iridology since 1983 and is the author of *The Integrated Iridology Textbook*.

expertise, and commitment to empowering individuals on their journey toward optimal health and well-being. Readers will undoubtedly find themselves captivated by the transformative potential of this ancient art and science.

It is nearly 20 years since this book was first published. In that time, I would have to say, iridology itself has probably not changed very much, if at all: so why is an update necessary or desirable?

Speaking personally, as its author, I would have to say it breaks down to two main reasons.

The first is that the original, while fairly complete in its own right, still omitted material that I did originally submit, but which, for reasons that seemed good at the time, were cut from the final manuscript. Among these, the chapter on the diatheses—the third level of constitutional analysis—has been reinserted, alongside "constitution" (color) and "disposition" (structure). Of all the generic constitutional iris indicators, diathesis is perhaps of the greatest assistance to Natural Healing, in that it invokes very specific treatment protocols and approaches, especially regarding detoxification. It was present to some extent in the original volume in the chapter on "The Iris and Its Signs." It has now been given its own chapter. In this regard, the constitutional descriptors themselves have, throughout the three levels of analysis, also been further expanded and developed.

Fresh material has also been inserted in the introductory chapters, specifically the notes on the derivation of the iris itself and its anatomical structure; a section emphasizing the importance of an understanding of terrain theory in iridology; and expanded notes on the methodology of holistic iris analysis. These, I believe, provide a more in-depth foundation for the understanding of the practice, commensurate with my own reading of the cultural sophistication of those I would like to reach, whether the interested individual or the professional iridologist.

The second reason for the new edition is that, irrespective of whether iridology has evolved substantially in the last twenty years, I have. My understanding and experience of the significance of the human iris has deepened beyond measure in that time. Consequently, there are things that I might express rather differently this time around, with fresh perspectives that are, I believe, important to emphasize. In this respect it is not so much a complete rewrite that has been necessary, but more a judicious change of emphasis here and there, sometimes quite subtle, that will recruit language to more precise levels of articulation.

Indeed, the articulation of iridology itself as a linguistic project—one in which the choice of words itself can make the difference between a superficial description of one's health tendencies and a penetrating analysis that ultimately returns all the parts to the whole in an integrated portrait of the individual—is itself an innovation that rests on significant paradigmatic revision, and one to which I devote considerable attention in the classroom and in professional practice. This I have tried to achieve in this revised, expanded edition of a book that has otherwise stood the test of time extremely well.

July 2023

Iridology is the examination and analysis of the colored portion of the eye—the iris—in order to determine factors that may be important in the prevention and treatment of disease, as well as in the attainment of optimum health.

One of the advantages of iridology is that it can reveal many aspects of an individual's health. An iris picture may suggest that where there is a problem, more than one organ may be involved, or that some emotional or mental element exists. This can lead to more appropriate advice being given, with the person having a choice of treatments, such as seeing a chiropractor or a naturopath.

My training was in the School of Natural Healing—a school of herbal medicine based on the European herbal tradition and the native North American healing arts founded by Dr. John Raymond Christopher. Dr. Christopher stopped at nothing in his efforts to heal sickness and to promote health, and his reputation for achieving success in cases of almost hopeless severity is legendary to this day. The book *The School of Natural Healing* is a classic of herbal literature and a compendium of natural, noninvasive healing techniques.

The three basic principles of Natural Healing are *simplicity*, *responsibility*, and *change*. The simplest idea in healing is that you don't have to heal your body, or get doctors and specialists to do so. Your body heals itself, naturally and effortlessly; it is precisely designed to repair and heal, and if it didn't, you would not survive. Natural Healing is the affirmation of the body's power to heal itself. However, it also recognizes that for healing to happen, you must assume responsibility for yourself and make appropriate adjustments in your life.

There are many different methods and styles of medicine available today, but the only true healer is Nature. The suggestions that you will find in this book are based on this premise. Therefore, instead of inorganic supplements, you will find foods; instead of drugs, you will find herbs; and instead of sophisticated specialist techniques, you will find commonsense suggestions that anyone can apply.

Iridology affirms the uniqueness of each individual and the power of the individual to manage his or her own health. Your eyes belong to you, and the information they hold is yours. Even if you consult a professional iridologist, you need to understand and resonate with the information you are given. It should have meaning for you and be understandable in the context of your life. Knowledge, in this case, is the power to help and heal yourself.

Today there are physicians and healers of many traditions and disciplines, including herbalists, homeopaths, and medical doctors, working with iridology. It is my hope that, as you progress through the book, you will begin to share in the fascination of discovery through looking at your own eyes.

2004

1

What is iridology?

Around the pupil of each of your eyes is a structure for which conventional science has, as yet, no full explanation. In our terms, it is a recognized indicator of heredity, differentiated primarily by color: the iris (plural: irides, pronounced "eye–rid–eez").

The eyes and the skin surrounding them are indicators of a variety of personal factors. We can infer that someone's health and vitality is below par if his or her eyes are tired, bloodshot, or lackluster, or if there are dark circles underneath them; conversely, a sparkle in someone's eyes can show laughter, joy, or love.

From the earliest epoch of human civilization, the eyes have been used to impart information about their owners. The Chinese discerned health tendencies from the size, shape, and set of the eyes, and in the Indian Ayurvedic tradition eye color and size is also part of a person's *Prakriti*, or constitution.

A PATHWAY TO GOOD HEALTH

Your irides are unique to you. Among the more than seven billion human inhabitants on Earth, not one has irides identical to yours: not just the colors, but the myriad structural variations that can be viewed in each iris—and they are not even the same as each other—are genetically determined evidence of your uniqueness.

It is estimated that some 200 differentiating signs may be charted in the irides, and bio-identification using the iris has been deployed at border controls, cash machines, and other access and security points. Iris identification works by noting the distribution of distinguishable characteristics—striations, pits, filaments, rings, freckles, darkened areas—within the eye's colored portion. Your irides offer some ten times greater security of identification than do your fingerprints.

> In Greek mythology, Iris was the goddess of the rainbow, who brought the messages of the gods to humanity. The full spectrum of the rainbow's colors is symbolic of the diversity of humankind and reflects the great variety of shades that occur in this portion of our anatomy.

A holistic methodology

Iridologists believe that treatment and lifestyle strategies for individuals must be based on an accurate assessment of the whole person and the factors that have shaped their lives. Hippocrates, the "father of modern medicine," said, "It is more important to know what sort of person has a disease, than to know the disease a person has."

Iridology has, at its heart, the humanistic and holistic traditions of medicine and healing, in which the integrity of the whole person is observed and honored. It has been, from its inception, a science that had more in common with the holistic, whole-person practices of natural and traditional healing methods than with mainstream medicine, with which, due to its symptom-based approach, it has always had a somewhat uneasy coexistence. This is reflected in its history and in the experiences of some of its most celebrated protagonists—a situation that continues to a large extent into the present day.

For example, online commentaries dealing with iridology are these days ever more subject to "editing" to downplay its validity and to cast aspersions upon those who practice it. My own experience, however, is that once medical professionals truly *understand* it, they are always fascinated and impressed, and I have taught this technique to many medical doctors.

Iridology depends only upon the examination of the irides:

sophisticated scientific equipment or testing procedures are unnecessary. All that is required is an ordinary magnifier, a flashlight, and sufficient knowledge to begin your interpretation.

Technical options, such as digital photography and slit-lamp bioscopes, certainly enhance the practice, but they are not strictly essential. Once you know how to handle a "torch and lupe," you can easily practice anywhere.

One of the questions that I am most commonly asked at the beginning of a consultation is, "Are you going to tell me what's wrong with me?" I am in the habit of answering such a question by saying, "I am just as likely to tell you what's RIGHT with you." People are sometimes genuinely afraid that they will be diagnosed with some hitherto unsuspected disease, and, indeed, if iridology can be said to be dangerous, it would be because of its potential to activate the *nocebo* effect.

Nocebo: from Latin *nocere*, to harm or hurt. The so-called nocebo effect is a play on the placebo effect, where an inert medicine is found to work just as well as the real thing because patients believe they are being treated. Nocebo is the insertion of a negative idea, which has a similarly powerful effect—but to the detriment of the patient.

Early in my career I developed the practice of ensuring that my first comment upon examining the iris bore a positive message. It is much better to begin with some encouraging words to set expectations of relaxation, self-discovery, and healing. To help you, if you are a beginner, as we go through the basic iris types, we give examples of positive messages that can be given for each type.

A critical part of the methodology used in iridology assessment is that we generally do not make hard-and-fast assertions until we have conducted a thorough investigation. Even then, in terms of actual pathology, we are unlikely to "diagnose" the way we would expect our GP to do it: we recognize that the actual identification of a "real pathology" needs to be conducted by experts in that particular field, with equipment to which generally only they have access—such as laboratories, scanning machines, surgeries, and so forth.

As iridologists, we are far more interested in the underlying conditions that are the causes of chronic or serious health problems than we are in the simple naming of diseases. Therefore, rather than tell someone, for example, that she may be "prediabetic," we will discuss her taste preferences (cravings for sweet foods), ask about any tendency toward symptoms when hungry (feeling nauseous or irritable), her digestive functions in general, and her family history, and then we proceed to giving practical advice designed to prevent the development of a named disease state and reverse any perceived tendency in that direction.

One of my teachers once said: the skill of an iridologist is to know the right questions to ask. This practice of using *questioning* to verify the observations from the irides is central, and it also gets us out of trouble. There was once an iridology lecturer who scared the life out of his students when he walked into a classroom, pointed at each in turn, and said words like, "arthritis," "IBS," "anxiety," "autoimmunity," and even "cancer." No such assumptions can *ever* be made, and no matter what is in your irides, the message has to be one of hope and positivity: you do not have to be ill, no matter what your irides appear to say. Nothing is written in stone, and

Using an iriscope

When you have an iridology consultation, one of the procedures the iridologist will perform is to study your eyes and irides using a specially set up digital camera (Figure 1.1). This creates photographs of your eye, and these can be easily and quickly mounted on a computer screen and used to explain the practitioner's diagnostic process.

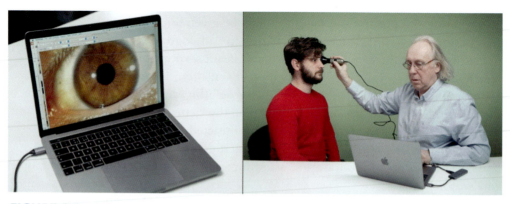

FIGURE 1.1.

Using an iriscope.

what is written in the iris is simply a map of possibilities. *You* get to determine whether you activate those tendencies or not, and, if you already have, the task of the iridologist is, first, to explain how it happened and then to advise you what you need to do to reverse that detriment.

This procedural etiquette in iridology is very important, and it encompasses one of the main theoretical foundations of the method: we may see signs and markings in the irides that are suggestive of "diseases," but, in actual fact, what those signs are pointing to is the underlying dynamic out of which what we call the "disease" may arise. The questions that we ask will be aimed at ascertaining whether, or to what extent, those disease possibilities are active, or whether they remain latent. Once this is understood, we can begin to offer practical, individualized advice toward reversing or rebalancing those tendencies.

Conventional diagnosis

At its simplest level, diagnosis means to determine the nature of a disease through examination of the indications. These indications include the symptoms reported by the individual as well as both visible and hidden signs. A visible sign might be something about the person that gives you a clue, such as posture, skin color, facial expression, tongue, pulse, odor, or vocal characteristics. Hidden signs are usually the result of changes in blood chemistry, hormone levels, and internal tissues. Modern medicine has developed a range of tests, from simple urine and blood analyses to surgical tissue sampling, endoscopy, and scanning procedures such as echocardiogram and ultrasound, CAT, and MRI scans, to discover such changes.

Complementary health practitioners are increasingly being taught *differential diagnosis*, which enables them to make the same *initial* assessments as medical doctors (GPs), through observing and recording symptoms, performing a physical examination, taking blood pressure, or palpating (examining through touch), and then determining which disease or condition fits the indications best.

These diagnostic methods are, however, all *disease-oriented* and probably conclude with the doctor/practitioner saying, "I think you have such-and-such a condition," then selecting a treatment to combat the assumed "disease." But how useful is this diagnosis to you? Does it empower you to tackle the problem? Sometimes a diagnosis can result in fear and depression, as we struggle with the shock of hearing the seriousness of our condition (nocebo).

Prognosis

Alongside a medical diagnosis, we also may be given a prognosis: what is the likely development and outcome of the disease with or without treatment? In this we are entirely in the hands of the experts, and we usually have no choice but to believe what they tell us, which may not be what we want to hear. What power do we have to influence or change that prediction?

If you think about it, a prognosis is only valid if you fit the usual profile of a disease sufferer: someone who does not know how to maximize his or her potential for vibrant health or take responsibility for turning things around. In fact, medical experience is peppered with stories of individuals who have disproved or outlived their prognosis through sheer determination and positive, creative, self-healing energy—or activation of the vital healing force that resides in all of us.

Similarly, in the history of medicine Hippocrates noticed more than 2,000 years ago that the same "disease" in two different people might have two different outcomes: one may suffer mildly and come through to regain full health; the other might even die. What makes the difference? Part of the answer is *individual constitution*.

With that in mind, let's propose a "prognosis equation" that can work for a variety of situations and individuals.

The prognosis equation

Prognosis = diagnosis + individual constitution + current health status + treatment chosen.

If you change any of the factors in a predictive equation, the outcome will be different. This way we can see that imprisoning a "patient" in a rigid diagnosis/prognosis that does not admit individual conditions, or often even the possibility of healing itself, is probably not going to be helpful.

Constitutional assessment

Some natural health practitioners and doctors have indeed realized that a disease-orientated process is not enough: lifestyle consider-ations, for example, have become increasingly important factors in determining health. But it also matters that each individual has his or her own unique constitution, which also has a role to play in determining the outcome of the situation.

This is where iridology plays a very specific and all-important part: it gives you a readout of your constitution, your essential makeup. This constitution outlines to a large extent your health predispositions, not as predictions written in stone, but as guide-lines to your body's innate mode of response. Iridology may also provide you with clues as to how your constitution has been affected by the choices and conditions of your life.

Constitution is assumed to be genetic: we can all probably think of problems our parents or grandparents had and then realize that there, but for the grace of God, we might also go—diseases "running in the family," and so forth. But we also acknowledge that perhaps, if we avoid some of the risk factors for that disease, we might *not* get the disease in the first place.

This leaves room for the concept of *epigenetics*: the degree to which our genetically inherited constitution can adapt, for better or for worse, to the conditions that it finds in its environment. In these terms its "environment" includes the diet that you feed it, the stresses that you expose it to, the lifestyle that you lead, and so on and so forth. In traditional European medicine (humoral medicine), this concept was known as the *Six Non-Naturals*:

1. Ambient air
2. Food and drink
3. Exercise and rest
4. Sleep and wakefulness
5. Retention and evacuation of wastes
6. Perturbations of the mind and emotions

The important thing to realize about *all* of these aspects of life is that they are all open to influence and *change*: you can do something about them. This means that if something is putting pressure on your natural constitution such that it starts to express symptoms, you can, by understanding your body's response, make relevant changes to put things back on track. In this it is also crucial that we realize that what we call *disease* is usually merely the effects caused by *our body's attempt at a healing or corrective response.*

These symptoms, therefore, are *not* the disease: they are evidence that the body has noted the adverse conditions and is attempting to do something about them. The body will *always* act to adapt and compensate—to heal itself, in fact. The symptoms are, therefore, the evidence of the same vital healing force that we have talked about. So many times in our culture these important signs are mistaken for the actual disease and suppressed with medication or with surgery. There are no exceptions to this rule: there is only the need to understand the individual case and work out what the body in its wisdom is trying to accomplish, and why.

A blueprint for wellbeing

This is more than diagnosis. To know the pathway to possible sickness is also to know the route out of it—or, indeed, the way to avoid it altogether.

It is generally accepted that if you eat sensibly, exercise moderately, give up harmful habits such as smoking and excessive drinking, and manage your stress levels, you are statistically likely to live a longer and healthier life. However, when deciding how to improve your lifestyle, you need to know what is healthy *for you*, as different factors affect people in different ways. In order to do this, you need a method to assess your unique requirements, and this must be based both on your current health status and on your genetically inherited constitution. This is where iridology comes in, as a uniquely individual assessment technique.

Iridology makes crucial information available to you—we might say, using marketing terms, your *strengths, weaknesses, opportunities,* and *threats* (SWOT). With this information you can make effective decisions about your health. It is just as vital for individuals, if they want to get well and stay well, to assess their positive characteristics as it is for them to be aware of their weaknesses and threats. The negative factors will advise caution in specific key respects. The positive factors will be allies that can be relied upon along the way.

Positive factors may also tell us something about our path in life, what work we are most suited to, what we look for in our relationships, and how we seek satisfaction. All of these factors are vital in determining what changes we need to make in order to reverse ill health. People who exacerbate their weaknesses and ignore their strengths will not be healthy or happy.

Using iridology, you are enabled to opt for a preventive health-care strategy: being aware of the potential for difficulties, you take preemptive evasive action. If you become aware of and respect your weaknesses, you may thus turn them into strengths, and so also convert potential threats to opportunities.

IRIDOLOGY TODAY

Iridology is one of a few disciplines that use the eye in a diagnostic capacity. Optometrists, for example, are able to identify a number of diseases by examining the interior of the eye. Doctors are aware of some of the signs recognized in iridology, particularly those relating to certain appearances in the cornea, which is one of the outer, transparent layers of the eye. Sclerology is another technique for evaluating health, in this instance through signs that appear in the whites of the eyes. Like iridology, with which it is linked, it also is largely the province of natural health practitioners.

In Europe, until fairly recently, iridology was actually taught in some medical schools—in Russia, for example, as late as 2000—and was informed by research conducted in medical contexts. The true picture of international iridology is that the different strands are now being woven into one. With excellent, dedicated researchers on every continent, iridology may now be poised to break through the prejudices that have surrounded it and take its place alongside more widely known medical disciplines.

Iridology is well established in many countries as a naturopathic health assessment technique. Due to its special characteristics, it has the potential to cross boundaries specified by the modern insistence upon "evidence-based" science. From the detailed physiology of the medical model, through the vitalistic approach of the naturo-pathic schools, to the broad-ranging skills of holistic practitioners, iridology has something to offer to everyone who is interested in discovering the underlying dynamics of health and disease.

Iridology is also highly useful in assessing the *potential* for toxic loading of body tissues, leading to specific advice regarding detoxification protocols that may need to be applied. This renders it especially useful to naturopaths, who believe that it is only possible to build good health on a clean and balanced terrain. In fact, it could, with some justification, be said that an iridology assessment is indeed an assessment of the terrain, in the sense that biochemist Pierre Jacques Antoine Béchamp [1816–1908] used that term to describe the underlying condition of the body that gives rise to what we, in our modern medical era, refer to as "infections," which are widely regarded as the activities of supposedly disease-causing microbial organisms.

Terrain theory vs. germ theory

Béchamp, along with his contemporary, physiologist Claude Bernard [1813–1878], hypothesized that the tissue status of the individual is crucial in determining its operational functionality and its ability to either support or undermine the health of the individual organism. In fact, Bernard's concept of the *milieu intérieur* ["internal environment"] is widely regarded as the forerunner of the currently accepted biomedical notion of *homeostasis*: the complex range of biochemical processes that produce a dynamic equilibrium in which *biological systems maintain stability while continually adjusting to external and internal conditions.*

There is a substantial contemporary movement to reestablish "terrain theory" in opposition to the current adherence in medicine to "germ theory," which may be regarded as the combined brainchild of Louis Pasteur [1822–1895] and Robert Koch [1843–1910]. Germ theory won the day, largely due to strong financial support from industrialists of the day who were moving into the medical sector due to the profitability of selling pharmaceuticals, many of which are, still to this day, created out of the byproducts of the petrochemical industry. A comprehensive and thought-provoking history and analysis of germ theory can be found in William P. Trebing's ground-breaking book, *Good-Bye Germ Theory*.[1]

It is worth noting that the eminent nineteenth-century researcher Rudolph Virchow [1821–1902], regarded as the "Father of Pathology" for his discovery of cellular pathology as the underlying element in producing disease, reportedly declared that if he could relive his life, he would dedicate it to proving that diseased tissue is the preferred habitat of germs, rather than germs being the cause of diseased tissue.

Naturopathy, a discipline the roots of which can be traced back thousands of years, into antiquity, has long held that maintaining cleanliness and balance in lifestyle is the best route to reestablishing and perpetuating good health. In our time, naturopathy is currently in the flush of a reawakening in people's lives as we struggle with an unrelenting onslaught of toxic substances—most often the products of the very industrial processes that have, indirectly and directly, given us the pharmaceutical industry itself, which has profited so massively from germ theory.

This onslaught has flooded us with an almost inescapable diet of poor-quality, indigestible foods, and a stupendous range of environmental and atmospheric biotoxins, including chemicals never before encountered by the human immune system, and heavy metals, which are known disruptors of normal neurological, endocrine, and immune-system physiology. Most naturopaths, including myself, are continually faced with the ravaging effects of this and with the desperate, mounting need to detoxify our patients from all of this before ever they have a hope of being truly well.

In this endeavor, the iris and its secrets are invaluable indicators of the level of risk represented by such conditions. Although it is necessary to emphasize that the vast majority of what we see in the iris is not open to change or development as life progresses and does not alter visibly according to the conditions the organism meets in life (either positively or negatively), there do exist examples of what we might call acquired accumulations of health-disrupting material. These become visible as the person ages—one of these being the corneal sign that relates to high cholesterol and the possibility of ischemic circulatory disease. (See "The Cholesterol Ring: Lipemic Diathesis," in Chapter 5.)

More than this, however, the ability to assess the inherent strength and vitality of the body's inbuilt organs and systems of detoxification and elimination—the bowel, the liver, the kidneys, the lymphatic tissue, the skin—will determine the likely levels of accumulation and intoxication, given the individual's health history and trajectory, and is crucial in determining the pathways that will need to be cleared and reactivated in order to reverse the condition.

Iridology and the mind

The study of the iris has also entered the realm of the psyche. In fact, from the work of researcher Josef Deck[2] (see below), the idea that the genetic reality of the individual includes both somatic (body-orientated) and psychic (mind-orientated) phenomena can clearly be seen and understood, particularly in Deck's delineation of iris disposition (the *structural* components of any individual iris— see Chapter 4) in predicting certain typical or preprogrammed *behavioral* responses to the conditions encountered in life. That, by the way, is not to say that we cannot escape that preprogramming, which is simply adaptation in another form, but we have to become conscious and aware of it.

Later contributions, such as those by researchers Denny Ray Johnson,[3] Harri Wolf, Daniele Lo Rito, Jim Verghis,[4] and Toni Miller,[5] have moved closer to a humoral theory of health and disease linked to individual psychological and emotional experience, in which the iris is the focus of a holistic analysis of the multidimensional field of human awareness.

This is very much in tune with vitalistic and energetic health models such as the Greco–Roman tradition, traditional Chinese medicine (TCM), and Ayurveda. In these models there is no strict dividing line between mind and body, such a concept having arisen as a specific feature of post-Cartesian European philosophy. The ancients did not recognize such a demarcation or partitioning of the individual: mental, emotional, and physical phenomena all arose out of the constitution of the individual, which was regarded as the entirety of a person's being.

In terms of naturopathy, it is also long recognized that it is not just the physical, but the totality of a person—body, mind, and spirit—that must be attended to in "treatment." Once understood correctly, the iris may, in this context, serve as a guide to a person's inner reality, as well as the "outer" reality of bodily illness. (A detailed exposition of this layer of iris analysis is for another volume; there are, however, references to character-related assessments in Chapter 4, as well as a brief introduction to the iris and its signs in Chapter 7.)

HISTORY AND PIONEERS OF IRIDOLOGY

It is not possible to say exactly where or when the practice of diagnosis through the eyes began. We suspect that the ancient Egyptians knew something of iridology, because in the Cairo museum there is a display of painted ceramic eyeballs, complete with detailed markings on the iris and sclera (whites of the eyes).

Iridology in Europe

In the seventeenth and eighteenth centuries, two European texts appeared: *Chiromatica Medica,* by Philippus Meyens, published in 1670, which makes reference to reflex sites in the iris, and *De Oculo et Signo* ("The Eye and its Signs"), by Christian Haertels, published in 1786. But there was still no coherent theory or practice of iridology.

The story of modern iridology really begins, however, in the nineteenth century, with a Hungarian physician called Ignácz von Péczely.

Ignácz von Péczely, Hungary [1826–1911]

The story goes that at the age of 11, the young Ignácz tried to free an owl that was trapped in a hunter's snare, and in the process the bird's leg was broken. He took the bird home to splint the leg and nurse it back to health. As he did so, he noticed a dark mark in a part of the bird's iris. Thinking that this was unusual, he continued to observe the phenomenon after the owl reportedly made the boy's garden its home following successful healing. Von Péczely was struck how, over the passage of time, 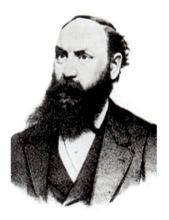 the mark changed to a paler shade, as though it was a record of a past trauma now healed.

In adulthood, von Péczely is said to have saved his mother's life with homeopathic remedies; as a result, people started to seek his help as a physician. He began to study the eyes of his patients, making correlations between their illnesses and the markings he observed, and achieved great renown for his seemingly magical ability to read a person's health from the eyes.

This soon attracted attention from the authorities, and an eminent physician accused von Péczely of fraudulent practice. He responded by peering intently into the man's eyes and giving him an on-the-spot diagnosis, which was so accurate that the doctor withdrew his allegations.

Von Péczely was aware that there would inevitably be further

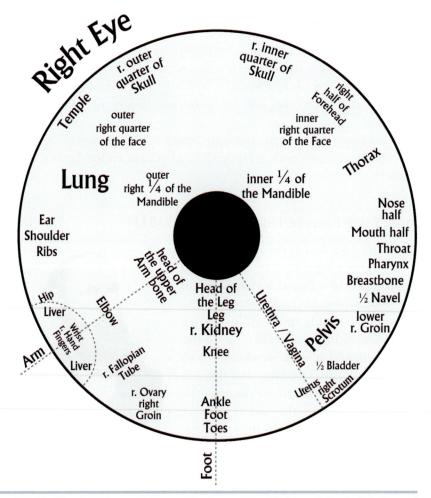

FIGURE 1.2

Ignatz von Péczely's Iris Chart. Enlarged irides with signs of the Right and the Left halves of

skirmishes, so he resolved to train as a medical doctor. This enabled the initial development of iridology as a medical science, as it gave von Péczely the opportunity to study the eyes of live patients and of cadavers, and to link postmortem findings with iris markings. In this way, he was able to conduct a huge amount of research, which forms the basis of the body of knowledge we now possess, as well as providing us with the first attempt at an iris chart (see Figure 1.2). Von Péczely's new system of diagnosis from the iris was first brought to the attention of the wider world through the writings of Emil Schlegel (*The Eye Diagnosis of I. V. Peczely*, 1886). He also published his own research in 1880 in *Discoveries in the Realm of Nature and Art of Healing.*

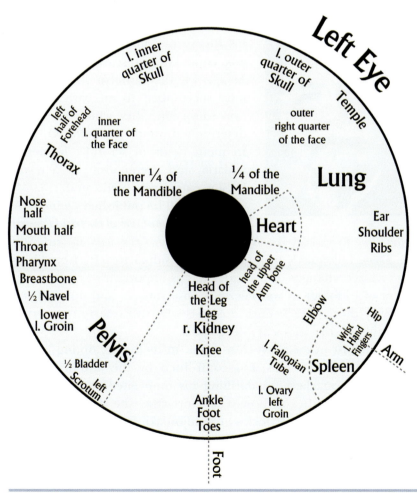

the body. The major organ positions in von Péczely's chart remain valid to this day. [l = left; r = right]

In the latter years of his career, von Péczely noticed that signs in the iris were not always accompanied by obvious ill health, and he struggled to understand why this was. His deathbed articulation of this conundrum—"*Hic signum, ubi ulcus?*" [Here's the sign, but where is the disease?] survives apocryphally to this day as the foundational question for contemporary iridology. It was resolved some decades later, when German researcher Josef Deck hypothesized that much of what is seen in the eyes is not the disease itself, but the genetic predisposition to disease: it is this understanding that forms the basis of iridology as we know it today.

Nils Liljequist, Sweden [1851–1936]

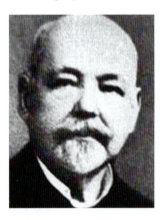

While Ignácz von Péczely developed his theory of iridology, Nils Liljequist was conducting research in Sweden. At age 14, the hitherto robust young man succumbed to an early vaccination campaign, after which his health deteriorated, and he suffered from frequent bouts of scrofula, influenza, malaria, and rheumatism; as a result, he was extensively medicated.

At age 20 he published *Quinine and Iodine Change the Color of the Iris: I Formerly Had Blue Eyes, They Are Now of a Greenish Color with Reddish Spots in Them*. Liljequist's hypothesis that residual toxicity from drugs had caused changes in his irides was as important to the development of iridology as von Péczely's observations, and up until very recently there have been iridologists who still referred to certain markings in the irides as "drug spots."

Liljequist never pursued a career in medicine, opting instead for the clergy. He was also confronted by the authorities and accused of quackery, establishing his innocence and reclaiming his reputation after a three-year court case, the details of which are recorded in Josef Deck's ground-breaking textbook on iridology, *The Principles of Iris Diagnosis*. Liljequist published his work, *Om Oegendiagnosen* [Diagnosis from the eye] in 1893. It contains a magnificent heritage of highly detailed drawings of irides, produced before the introduction of close-up photography.

Leopold Erdmann Emanuel Felke, Saxony [1856–1926]

Like Liljequist, Felke was a clergyman who performed naturo-pathic healing in his spare time, and promoted iridology widely in Europe. Felke's healing practice included a healthy diet and outdoor exercise, a diet very low in meat, healing earth applications (he was called "the Clay Doctor"), and cold baths in outdoor zinc bathtubs. He was also interested in medicinal herbs and homeopathy, and he became known as the father of combination homeopathic remedies, after he deviated from Christian Friedrich Samuel Hahnemann's [1755–1843] precepts and began combining different substances in the treatment of chronic disease. Felke was responsible for introducing a generation of younger physicians to the practice of iridology, and the *Felke Institut*, named after him, is currently Germany's foremost publishing and training body in iridology.

Rudolph Schnabel, Germany [1882–1952]

Schnabel was originally a pupil of Felke, but he went on to study medicine at the University of Zurich. He was, however, excluded from the institution for writing his doctoral thesis on iridology, although the ban was later rescinded. He published his research under the title *The Eye as a Mirror of Health*. The discovery of the *Schnabel lacuna*, an iris sign, is attributed to him, and is significant not only for bearing the name of its discoverer, but for bearing the shape of the name's meaning—in German, *Schnabel* means "beak": the sign is shaped like the beak of a bird.

Josef Deck, Germany [1914–1990]

Josef Deck was a medical doctor who founded the prestigious iridology research institute in Ettlingen, Germany. Ground-breaking work included his classification of the constitutional types based on color and structure of the iris. Deck regarded the iris primarily as an indicator of genotype; he held that iris appearances represented inherent predispositions. In 1965 he published *The Principles of Iris Diagnosis*, which

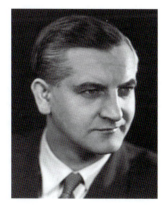

remains a cornerstone of iridology theory and has been heavily influential in almost all subsequent iridology textbooks, including this one, as well as *Information from Structure and Color* (2000), by Felke Institut writers, Willy Hauser, Josef Karl, and Rudolph Stolz.[6]

Joseph Angerer, Germany [1907–1994]

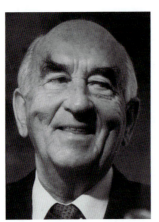

Joseph Angerer was a naturopath who originally studied iridology with Rudoph Schnabel and was also a colleague and close associate of Josef Deck. Angerer researched and developed one of the most detailed and accurate iris reflex charts; the many insights he presented have been definitive in the development of agreed iris topography and have found their way into the majority of contemporary iris charts, including the one offered by myself here in this book.

Iridology in America

Henry Edward Lane (early twentieth century)

Dr. Lane introduced iridology to the United States at the turn of the century, having emigrated from Austria. He was a medical doctor who carried out surgical and autopsy correlations with iris markings at the Kosmos Sanitarian in Evanston, Illinois, and published *Iridology: The Diagnosis from the Eye* in 1904.

Henry Lindlahr [1862–1924]

A student of Henry Lane, Dr. Lindlahr was also a medical doctor and osteopath. He turned to naturopathy after being helped by one of its forefathers, the famous Father Sebastian Kneipp [1821–1897] in Germany. Lindlahr published *Nature Cure: Philosophy and Practice* in 1913 and founded the ground-breaking journal, *Nature Cure*, in which several articles about iridology appeared, for the first time, in the United States. Lindlahr's work emphasized Natural Medicine and the so-called "healing crisis"—in the process of cleaning out accumulated toxins, the body may undergo a reactive crisis, whereby past illness and disease is partially reexperienced, and then released. He also warned of the dangers of suppressing symptoms. His book, *Iridiagnosis and Other Diagnostic Methods*, was published in 1922.

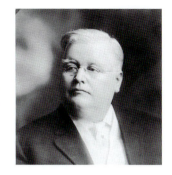

Bernard Jensen [1908–2002]

Dr. Jensen was arguably the most prolific and well-known naturopath in the twentieth century and the person who perhaps did more than any other single individual to put iridology on the global map. Originally a student of Lindlahr's, Jensen developed research on the "healing crisis." His promotion of bowel cleansing as foundational in naturopathic healing regimes is influential to this day, vindicated by much

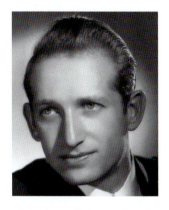

scientific research emanating from the functional medicine schools. He also qualified in chiropractic, osteopathy, nutrition, homeopathy, reflexology, and hydrotherapy. In 1982 he published *Iridology: The Science and Practice in the Healing Arts*,[7] among many other texts on iridology and naturopathy. His iridology reflex chart has been adopted as the standard for professionals in the twentieth and twenty-first centuries. I am personally fortunate and honored to have studied with Dr. Jensen briefly when he visited the United Kingdom in the late 1970s.

John R. Christopher [1909–1983]

Dr. Christopher, a friend and colleague of Bernard Jensen, is the author of *The School of Natural Healing*,[8] primarily a book on herbal medicine, which forms the philosophical and practical basis for the Association of Master Herbalists in the United Kingdom, of which I was a cofounder in 1995. Dr. Christopher's reputation rests particularly on his work with those suffering with supposedly incurable illnesses and conditions, but he was insistent that iridology as a diagnostic technique was invaluable in penetrating to the true underlying causes of the conditions he encountered in his patients. Dr. Christopher was a powerful influence on my own main teacher in herbal medicine and natural healing, Dr. Richard Schulze— also an iridologist.

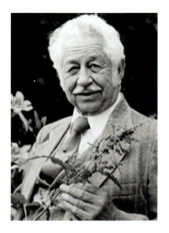

* * *

There have been many other pioneers and developers within the field of iridology, and it is not my intention to disrespect or discount any of them. Some—in particular Harri Wolf (United States) and Daniele Lo Rito (Italy)—have been my personal teachers and thus directly influential on my own work. In iridology, as elsewhere, we recognize that we stand on the shoulders of giants, some of whom do not necessarily command global status, but who have been, nonetheless, passionate teachers and interlocutors for iridology; without them, the practice could scarcely have survived.

NOTES

1. Trebing, W. P. (2019). *Good-Bye Germ Theory*. Author.
2. Deck, J. (1965). *Grundlagen der Irisdiagnostik* [The Principles of Iris Diagnosis]. Ettlingen: Josef Deck.
3. Johnson, D. R. (1995). *What the Eye Reveals*. Boulder, CO: Rayid.
4. Verghis, J. (2006). *Behavioural Iridology*. Mancos, CO: IM Publications.
5. Miller, T. (2021). *The Mind Matters: Emotional Aspects of Integrated Iridology*. Inter Health Australia Pty Ltd.
6. Hauser, W., Karl, J., & Stolz, R. (2000). *Information from Structure and Colour*. Heimsheim: Felke Institut.
7. Jensen, B. (1982). *Iridology, the Science and Practice in the Healing Arts*. Escondido, CA: Bernard Jensen Enterprises.
8. Christopher, J. R. (1976). *The School of Natural Healing*. Springville, IL: Christopher Publications.

2

The anatomy
of the eye and the iris

By looking at the eye anatomically, we can uncover some of the underlying rationale for iridology. We also can get close to a scientific explanation for the phenomena that form the basis of the observations made by the iridology pioneers.

According to iridology theory, the function of the iris involves far more than the conventional medical definition, which depends on the operation of the muscles of dilation and contraction, for the facilitation of sight. Like the fingertips, the iris is very rich in nerve supply. The fingertips are highly specialized for the sensation of touch, yet the iris itself is not normally considered to be a sensory organ.

Experiments have been conducted in which thin beams of light are directed at specific "reflex" sites in the iris, and the bodily organs that correlate to these sites on the reflex chart are assessed for degrees of stimulation. At this point in time, these experiments have not yet proven conclusive; in terms of the function and purpose of this complex innervation of a relatively simple anatomical structure, the jury is still out. Are there actual neurological connections—either anatomical or possibly involving chemical signaling—between iris sectors and the organs that they are said to reflect? Or are we perhaps looking at more of a holographic structure, in which the smallest anatomical part contains the information from which the whole system may be reconstructed?

Iridology is frequently seen as similar to reflexology or acupuncture in this respect, the iris representing an "energetic" blueprint that predicts what conditions would be encountered in the system thus represented. It is not, in fact, so far from the contemporary understanding of genetic conditions, which are understood to often contain codified information relating to the health risks of an individual. The research that might shed light on this, by comparing iridology findings to genetic profiles, has not yet, to my knowledge, been forthcoming. Such research would be time-consuming and fraught with ethical and method-ological difficulties, and in our culture of rigid scientific norms, funding is not generally available for any project containing the word "iridology". However, I am, as I write, in process of design-ing such a research program.

For now, let us focus on what we do know about the anatomy and physiology of the eye and its iris.

THE STRUCTURE OF THE EYE

The eye is a hollow sphere composed of a tough, fibrous material, the sclera, which is visible as the white of the eye (see Figure 2.1). The chamber of the eye is filled with a transparent fluid, or humor, known as vitreous jelly, through which light is conducted easily without distortion. At the back it is joined to the optic nerve, a stalk of nerve fibers issuing from the brain. This is the wiring that carries the signals received by the eye back to the seat of consciousness.

The optic nerve enters the eyeball and then spreads around its interior surface to form the retina. It is on the retina that the focused image of what we see is projected and then transferred through the optic nerve to the brain. The tissues of the optic nerve and the retina are continuous, and this has importance for iridology.

The retina contains specialized cells called rods and cones, which are photosensitive, allowing light to be captured and trans-mitted along nerve fibers. Human retinal cells are then further specialized in order to be able to register light of different wavelengths—that is, color.

Roughly opposite the junction with the optic nerve is an

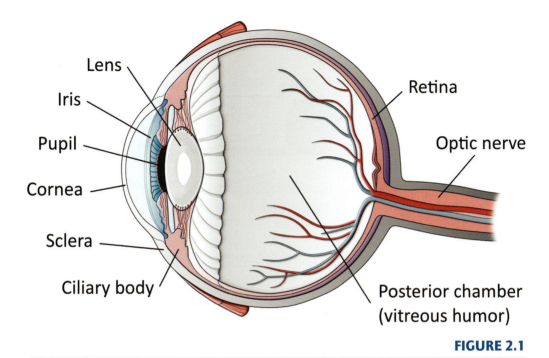

Lens

Iris

Pupil

Cornea

Sclera

Ciliary body

Retina

Optic nerve

Posterior chamber
(vitreous humor)

FIGURE 2.1

Anatomical diagram of the eye.

opening in the sphere of the eyeball: the pupil. This is the aperture
through which light and images enter, to register upon the retina.
Anchored to the edges of this opening are two structures vital to
sight: the lens and the iris.

The lens is a convex sliver of transparent tissue delicately
suspended behind the opening through which all light entering
the eye must pass, and which, like the lens of a camera, focuses the
image on the "photographic plate" of the retina. Muscles attached
to the eyeball enable the eye to focus. They alter the shape of the
chamber of the eye, and therefore the focal length of the signal.

A camera-like structure

The sensory cells of the eye are an extension of the brain, budding
out from the brain during fetal development. Like a camera, the
delicately suspended lens focuses the image on the retina, which
contains photosensitive cells.

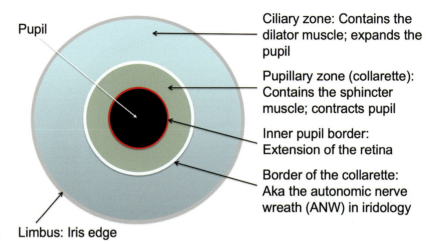

Pupil

Ciliary zone: Contains the dilator muscle; expands the pupil

Pupillary zone (collarette): Contains the sphincter muscle; contracts pupil

Inner pupil border: Extension of the retina

Border of the collarette: Aka the autonomic nerve wreath (ANW) in iridology

Limbus: Iris edge

FIGURE 2.2

Simple iris topography.

In front of the lens is the iris. The iris is a ring of connective tissue supplied with a musculature capable of contracting or expanding the size of the pupil, thereby regulating the amount of light that can enter the chamber (Figure 2.2). Immediately around the pupil is the sphincter muscle. Like other sphincters in the body, it is a ring muscle, the operation of which causes the pupil to contract, limiting the amount of light that can enter. The pupil should contract visibly if you shine a bright light into the eye.

In the outer portion of the iris are radial muscle fibers, which work to expand the pupil by pulling the inner edges outward. Our pupils naturally expand in poor light or darkness, so as to maximize the intake of light.

Checking your pupils

You can check the expansion and contraction of your pupils by shining a pen flashlight into the side of your eye, standing in front of a mirror.

▷ Flash the light repeatedly into one of your eyes, making sure that you are shining the light from the side of your eye and not directly into your pupil, which may cause some discomfort.

> ▷ Observe the changes in the size of your pupil. It will contract as you shine the light into it.
>
> ▷ When shining the light steadily into your eye, you will notice that, after a short interval, your pupil expands again as your eye becomes accustomed to the extra light. This expansion represents an automatic readjustment due to internal impulses from the nervous system.

The pupillary ruff, or inner pupil border (IPB)

The optic nerve, having entered the chamber of the eye, becomes the retina and forms a layer over the inner surface of the iris. This layer curls around the inner surface, behind the iris, and emerges as a fine, reddish-brown ruff around the edge of the pupil: the inner pupil border (IPB), or the *pupillary ruff*. This structure is important in iridology, as it can give information about the central nervous system.

Checking your pupillary ruff

In order to see your pupillary ruff, you will need a pen flashlight and a small magnifying glass; alternatively, you may wish to purchase a "self-examination mirror."

▷ Shine the light at your eye from the side, and look directly at your eye through the glass, or in the mirror, which should be held as close as necessary in order to maintain a sharp focus.

▷ The pupillary ruff is visible at the border of the inner edge of your iris and pupil. It appears as an uneven, segmented reddish-brown ring (Figure 2.3), and it is normal for the thickness of the ruff to vary around the ring.

▷ This minute ring is the visible extension of the tissue of the central nervous system, continuous with the retina and the optic nerve; it is the only place in the body where such tissue becomes accessible to sight.

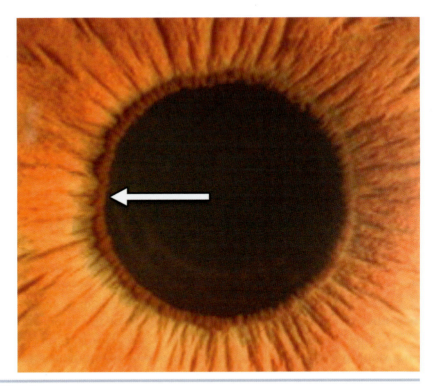

FIGURE 2.3

The inner pupil border.

THE STRUCTURE OF THE IRIS

The iris is a doughnut-shaped portion of muscle and connective tissue anchored to the shell of the eyeball at the *limbus*, or iris root, which is the visible outer edge of the iris. The muscles are contained in the deeper layers of the structure, but in front of these is the portion of the iris known as the iris body, or *stroma* (Figure 2.4).

The origin and development of the iris is to be found deep in the processes of growth and development of the individual, from embryonic life in the uterus through birth and beyond. Developing from a differentiated layer of cells in the embryo known as the *neuroectoderm*, the iris is, as its name suggests, a combination of both nerve and external, epithelial tissue. As we have seen, it is

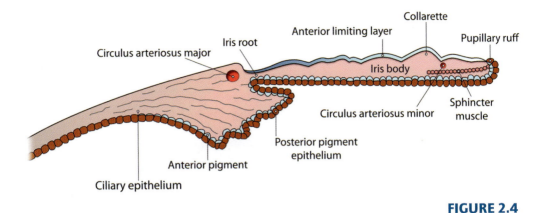

FIGURE 2.4

Cross-section of the iris.

also the only place where the tissue of the central nervous system can be seen directly with the naked eye.

The stroma

The stroma is a body of connective tissue, made up of thousands of very fine filaments. The filaments are arranged radially around the pupil in degrees of density, which vary greatly from one person to another and can also vary within the different sectors of each individual iris. It is the arrangement of these filaments, or *iris fibers*, which constitutes the "iris print." Each iris print is unique and is used by iridologists to assess inherent health and personality trends. The density of the layers of fibers is a factor in the assessment of constitutional strength, stamina, and resistance. (See Figure 2.5.)

The stroma of each iris also contains approximately 28,000 "blind" nerve endings. These nerves can be traced back to an area within the thalamus known as the lateral geniculate body. It is possible that here there are connections to all the organs and systems throughout the body; however, medical science has not yet offered a full explanation for this anatomical arrangement.

There are some four layers of fibers in the body of the iris; these can sometimes be seen clearly where there is an interruption in the density of the fiber structure (see below under "Crypts and Lacunae"). Within these fibers there also exists vascular tissue—in

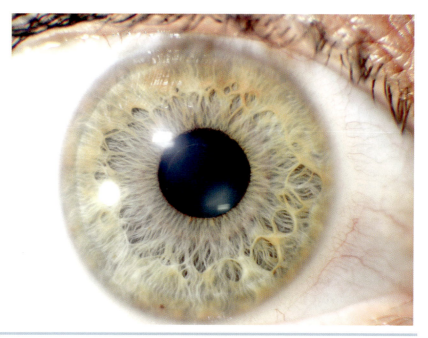

FIGURE 2.5

The fiber structure of the iris is highly individual.

fact, one older term used in anatomy and in iridology for this portion of anatomy of the eye is the "vascular arcade" (Figure 2.6). All tissue needs a blood supply, and the network of vessels that supports the iris includes both the major and the minor arterial circles.

Crypts and lacunae

Yet another name for this portion of the anatomy of the eye is the *crypt layer*, indicating the location of structural phenomena originally called *crypts of Fuchs* (after the Austrian ophthalmologist Ernst Fuchs [1851–1930]). Crypts are small holes in the iris stroma that allow through close microscopy something of a view into the interior of this fascinating and highly individual structure. They are significant in iridology according to their location, whereby they flag up potential organ weakness or loss of resistance. These "lesions" (as they are also called) can be of varying sizes, depths, and distributions. Occasionally they can pervade the entire iris, giving an impression of low fiber density (see "The Flexible–Adaptive Iris," in Chapter 4), and they are distinguishing features in the hormone- and digestive-regulatory dispositions.

In iridology, smaller openings, often having roughly symmetrical rhomboid shapes, are called *crypts* (see Figure 2.7), whereas larger structures, with a variety of typically more rounded shapes, are known as *lacunae* (Figure 2.8), which is the Latin plural of *lacuna*, meaning a small pool. (For a fuller discussion on the significance of crypts and lacunae, see Chapter 7.)

This complex structure of the stroma is not fully developed at birth. If you look into the eyes of a newborn baby, you may notice that his or her eyes are dark pools without differentiating features. In the weeks after birth, you can see some cloudy appearances beginning to form, the ghost of an emerging pattern until, at between three and four months of age, the iris, in terms of the precise layout of fibers and tissue structure, becomes fully formed.

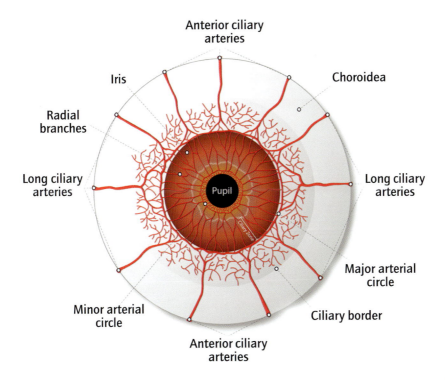

FIGURE 2.6

Vascularization of the iris.

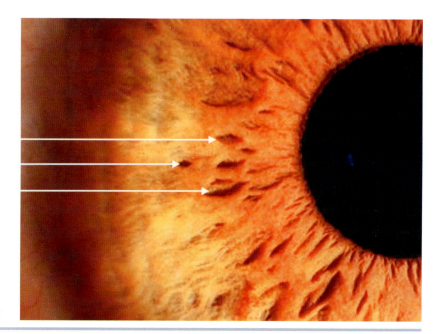

FIGURE 2.7

Crypts within the iris stroma.

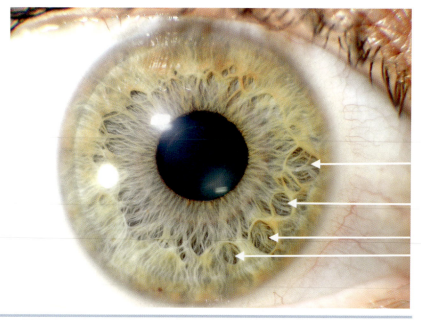

FIGURE 2.8

Lacuna structures within the iris.

Pigmentation may, however, continue to develop even up to the teenage years, although those born with the pure dark brown iris type (see Chapter 3) will be identifiable as such soon after birth.

Pigmentation

At the base of the stroma lies a layer of tissue known as the base leaf. This layer is pigmented a dark blue or charcoal gray and is considered to be the reason why blue eyes are blue. The fibers in blue eyes are actually whitish or pale gray, and the blue color is a reflection of the underlying base leaf through the fiber structure. Some research has suggested that this layer is receptive to light, and that a hole in the stroma (*lacuna*) permits the penetration of light to stimulate reflex sites deep in the iris, thus perhaps partly explaining the abovementioned phenomenon of the rich innervation of iris tissue.

The stroma also contains pigment-secreting cells that are responsible for brown eyes (Figure 2.9). The pigmentation from these cells is sometimes so dense—as in pure dark brown eyes—that

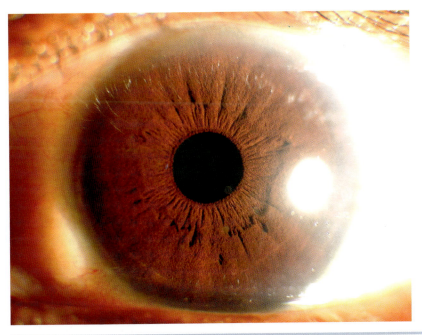

FIGURE 2.9

Fully pigmented dark brown iris.

the fibers that compose the iris cannot be seen. It is thought that the function of this pigment, like pigmentation of the skin, is to protect against strong sunlight, and therefore it displays an inherited adaptation to a hot climate. In blue eyes these cells appear to be largely dormant, and the blue iris type is thus considered to be "unpigmented."

Cornea, conjunctiva, and anterior border layer

The iris stroma is contained in its outer aspect by a thin transparent sheath—the anterior border layer—and then by the cornea and the conjunctiva, which are the outermost layers of the eye. The cornea is a transparent extension of the tough sclera (the word itself means "hard"), and the conjunctiva is a thin mucous membrane that not only covers the sclera and the cornea, but is also found lining the inside of the eyelids.

The anterior border layer and the cornea are important to iridology, as it is within these layers that some important iris signs are found. The cornea is the location of one of the best-known health-indicating eye signs: the corneal arcus or *arcus senilis* ("arc of old age") (Figure 2.10) and the corneal annulus (a white milky ring around the outer aspect of the iris), which is related to the possibility of high cholesterol, atherosclerosis, and ischemic vascular disease.

The anterior border layer is often found to contain pigment deposits known as "secondary pigments" (Figure 2.11) which can indicate disease-related metabolic issues such as enzyme deficiency and reduced capacity of detoxification mechanisms. (See a discussion of both these signs in Chapter 5.)

Autonomic nerve wreath (ANW)

If you look closely at an iris, you will see that it is divided into two concentric portions. Around the pupil, typically a third of the way out toward the edge of the iris, a roughly circular structure, which seems to project somewhat from the level of the rest of the iris, is usually evident. This is the autonomic nerve wreath (ANW) or the *border of the collarette* (BC)—the collarette being one of the names given to the inner circle immediately around the pupil and

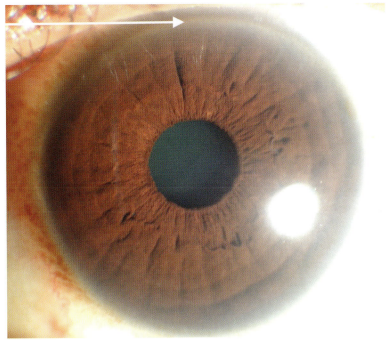

FIGURE 2.10

The arcus senilis in the cornea.

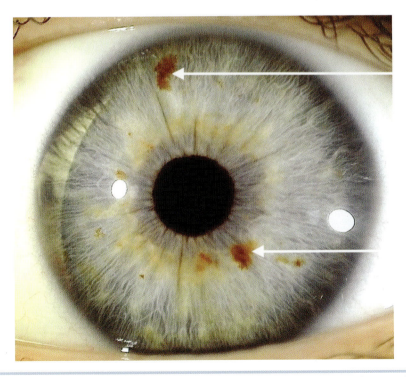

FIGURE 2.11

Secondary pigments in the anterior border layer.

inside the ANW, which, in the iridology reflex chart (see Bernard Jensen, Chapter 1), depicts the digestive tract.

Anatomically, the BC marks the position of the minor arterial circle (see Figure 2.6 above), and its appearance varies considerably from one individual to another. In some people it is invisible, while in others it is prominent and may appear jagged or serrated (see Figure 2.12). Occasionally, it may encircle the pupil closely and tightly, whereas in others it may reach out almost to the edge of the iris. In lighter colored eyes it is sometimes marked by a distinctly different color, known as a *central heterochromia*, which simply means "different color in the middle"; this may radiate out into the surrounding iris tissue. The meaning of this sign (discussed in Chapter 7) always relates to digestive function.

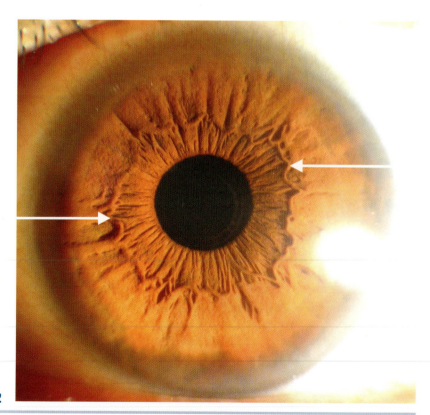

FIGURE 2.12

The border of the collarette.

The ANW reveals, as the name suggests, information about the autonomic nervous system (ANS), which is the part of the nervous system that runs the show, no matter what else you happen to be doing. So, for example, you don't have to remember to breathe, or to keep your heart beating: the ANS does that for you. But since in iridology it also represents the boundary between the digestive organs and the rest of the system, the ANW specifically refers to what anatomists have called the *enteric nerve system*—the specific nerve supply to the gastrointestinal tract.

Iridologists closely observe the variations, undulations, and degree of prominence of the ANW, which reveal nerve-supply issues affecting digestion, but also key individual tendencies in character, behavior, and temperament. To understand this, consider how many expressions we use that link feeling and emotion to the gut: the phrase "gut feeling" itself, or being unable to "stomach" something, or things that "make us sick."

The nerve supply to the iris

Two opposing muscle systems—the dilator and sphincter muscles—are housed in the iris; these control the size of the pupil through the operation of the ANS, which has two branches: the sympathetic nervous system (SNS) and the parasympathetic nervous system (PSNS). The dilator muscles of the iris are influenced mainly by the SNS, whereas the sphincter muscle is mainly powered by the PSNS.

The SNS is also called the "fight-or-flight" response. When you are under stress or are suffering from anxiety or shock, your pupils will tend to dilate. This is a physiological response designed to maximize the amount of information available to you at times of threat or danger. Nature knows that in difficult circumstances the slightest detail could be crucial to the preservation of life. (See Figure 2.13.)

The PSNS is, conversely, known as the "rest-and-digest" response. The main nerve in the parasympathetic system is the vagus nerve, which is largely responsible for the nerve supply to the gastrointestinal tract; it is this part of the nervous system that

Table 2.1   Sympathetic and Parasympathetic Nervous Systems

Organ response	Sympathetic system: "Fight or flight"	Parasympathetic system: "Rest and digest"
Eyes	Pupils dilate	Pupils contract
Heart	Heart rate accelerates	Heart rate slows
Lungs	Bronchi dilate	Bronchi contract
Stomach	Inhibits gastric acid	Stimulates gastric acid
Liver	Glucose release stimulated	Bile release stimulated
Intestines	Peristalsis & secretions inhibited	Peristalsis & secretions stimulated
Bladder	Relaxes / empties	Contracts / stores

needs to be dominant while your body is digesting food. This is why eating when you are stressed or upset should be avoided; if you are under the influence of the SNS, you will not digest your food well.

These two branches of the ANS are designed to counterbalance each other, so that the sympathetic nerves help us to respond appropriately to the demands of life, while the parasympathetic impulses ensure that, when the action is over, we are brought back to a calm and relaxed state. Some people may, however, become fixated in one mode—usually the sympathetic nerve response—characterized by states of high excitation or even anxiety—as though there is a constant threat to counter. Parasympathetic nerve dominance, on the other hand, may indicate a tendency toward sluggishness and lack of motivation.

Each of us has our default setting in this regard. To find out what this is, observe the size of the pupil: an enlarged iris and a "wide-eyed" look indicates an SNS-dominant person, inclined to fast responses, and consequently possibly at risk of exhaustion over time. A contracted and small iris, on the other hand, indicates a PSNS-dominant person who is slow to respond; she or he may, however, also be harboring inner tensions that are not obvious to the casual observer.

Assessing the size of your pupils

Studying the size of your pupils can give you a good idea of how your nervous system operates (see Figures 2.13 and 2.14).

Looking at your own eyes, try to estimate the relative size of your pupil in comparison to your eye.

- ‣ Shine a pen flashlight steadily into the side of your eye. Your pupil will contract. After a short interval, your pupil will expand again, as your eye becomes accustomed to the extra light. Remember, when shining the light into your eye, to let it linger long enough for the eye's initial light-sensitive reaction to subside.
- ‣ A normal proportion is for the radius of the pupil to be approximately one quarter of the radius of the iris.

These are general principles, and your pupil size may also change according to how you feel and what is happening in your life. You can monitor this over time in order to determine the normal size of your pupils.

Influences on autonomic nerve activity

Variation in pupil size also may occur with the use and abuse of certain drugs. Barbiturates, opiates, and other tranquilizers cause contraction of the pupils, whereas stimulating drugs such as cocaine, amphetamines, and hallucinogens like LSD character-istically result in wide-open pupils.

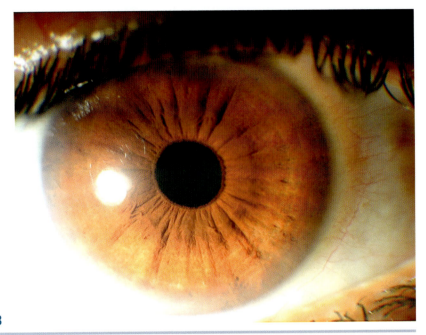

FIGURE 2.13

Small pupil: Parasympathetic dominance; slow to respond, risk of nervous tension

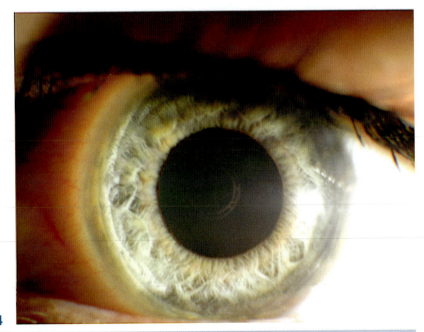

FIGURE 2.14

Large pupil: Sympathetic dominance; fast responses, risk of nervous exhaustion

Activators of sympathetic nerves:

▷ adrenaline, anxiety, fear, "fight-or-flight" situations, stress, exhilaration;

▷ drugs: ephedrine (used in bronchodilators), cocaine, LSD, cannabis and alcohol (first stage), amphetamines ("speed" or "uppers");

▷ withdrawal from opiates (compensatory reaction).

Effects upon physiology:

▷ pupils dilate, blood vessels contract, blood pressure and heart rate increase.

Activators of parasympathetic nerves:

▷ rest and relaxation, digestion, meditation, sleep, endorphin release after exercise;

▷ drugs: barbiturates, opiates, sleeping pills, benzodiazepines (e.g., Valium), "downers"; second stage of cannabis and alcohol use;

▷ herbal remedies: "nervines" (nerve-relaxants).

Effects upon physiology:

▷ pupils contract, blood pressure decreases, vessels dilate, heart rate slows.

Extrovert or "external processor"

If your pupils are habitually larger than one quarter of the radius of your iris, you are mostly under the influence of your SNS. You will tend to be active, outgoing, open and trusting, and enjoy the challenges of life. Your responses may well be spontaneous, if occasionally impulsive and reckless. If the enlargement is extreme, you may have a tendency to overactivity or overstimulation of the adrenal glands. This can be a prelude to exhaustion. You should assess your lifestyle and the demands you are making upon your body: you may be overworking or neglecting your own interests in favor of others', and you may need to draw firmer boundaries to contain and preserve your energy levels.

Introvert or "internal processor"

If your pupils are generally smaller than average, you are mostly under the influence of your PSNS. You may be slow to trust people, take your time to deliberate in making decisions, and are careful how you use your energy. You are, therefore, not as prone to depletion and exhaustion as the "open" type. However, with the parasympathetic nerves dominant, there may be a tendency toward a lack of motivation, too much sleep, and a lack of exercise. Think about ways in which you can redress this balance by becoming more physically engaged with the world.

DO IRIS FEATURES CHANGE?

There has been considerable debate in iridology circles around whether, or to what extent, iris features change, particularly as an indicator of the success or otherwise of treatment. The old idea that detoxification, specifically, can result in a clearance of pigmentation (either primary or secondary) has pretty much been debunked through an almost complete lack of photographic evidence. Stories of lacunae, or lesions, closing up or being "darned" by "healing fibers" have proved similarly unverifiable, with one notorious case where photographs were found to have been doctored in order to "prove" the hypothesis.

In fact, the iris is a remarkably stable structure, and beyond certain age-related changes (such as the so-called cholesterol ring) and the phenomenon of adolescent acquisition of second-ary pigments (see "The Dyscratic Overlay", in Chapter 5), what is observed in early life will still be present, and identical, in old age. Josef Deck felt that the iris was not fully developed until the age of 6 years. I personally am of the opinion, from my own observa-tions, that in some cases that timeline can be extended to the attainment of full adult maturity—or around the age of 18. After this, true iris change is rare, and would need careful assessment.

In many cases where changes are apparent, these can frequently be assigned to the phenomenon of pupil size changes: an expanded pupil will appreciably change the shape of lacunae by compres-sion of the iris tissue, making them appear rounder and fatter, whereas when the pupil contracts they will be drawn into a more linear and pointed formation. Similarly, the size of the pupil can greatly change the reflective potential of the iris, giving rise to apparent color changes. In this way, many reports of iris changes are actually the result of variations in pupil diameter from one examination to the next.

What this means for iridology is that claims that progress in treatment can be monitored by ongoing iris examination must be reassessed and discarded. Many are confused by this, as they feel that a diagnostic or assessment technique that cannot provide up-to-the-minute data is not useful. However, once you realize that the majority of the data that iridology provides is related to natal *constitution*, the conundrum is resolved, and the iris can take its true place as an indicator of the genetically inherited factors that underpin our health possibilities throughout life—for better or for worse.

3

The iridology constitutions: color types

Before we get to look at the iris chart, finding the signs and linking these to organs and systems, we need an overview of the individual body system and its characteristics and susceptibilities. This is to be found in the notion of constitution. Your constitution is unique to you, but in practice we find repeating patterns, or types, that can give us the ballpark before we go on to refine our search for the individual features.

"Constitution" is defined as the sum of your inherited and acquired characteristics, and it depends on two main factors. The first is genetic material encoded in DNA, which governs such characteristics as gender, height, skin and eye color, and the second is acquired experience—first in the uterus and then throughout life.

While the general understanding of genetic constitution is thought to depend on inherited traits from the parents, it is also possible that a major influence on iris development occurs *in utero*. The work of Swedish geneticist and embryologist Matts Larssen[1] has linked these two possibilities and shed some light on the processes involved, which appear to be linked to the regulatory influence of the PAX6 gene—a gene unique to sighted creatures, and one that is also known to be formative in terms of individual psychological response, especially regarding character or temperament, highlighting for us once again the close links between "body" and "mind." Your iris constitution may give us useful information not just about your organs and systems, but also about your personality and typical mode of being in the world.

In iridology, constitution is divided into three levels of assessment: *basic* or *primary constitution*, assessed by color; *disposition*, assessed by the structural variations affecting the iris fibers and their layout; and *diathesis*, which, for simplicity, I have termed the "overlay": the presence of additional material or accumulations in the iris. Of these three, the first two—primary constitution and disposition—are considered to be entirely inherited and not susceptible to apparent visual change; of the third—diathesis or overlay—two types are considered inherited, and two acquired.

The three levels are dealt with separately, in turn, in the following three chapters, but they are, in fact, always combined in the individual. This means that when giving an iridology "reading," it is important to identify each level in turn and assess its impact on the individual's health patterns, and then to put them all together as a holistic description of the totality of that person's health predispositions.

CONSTITUTION BY COLOR: OVERVIEW

There are three primary constitutional iris types defined by color. These consist of the two "pure" colors—blue and dark brown—and the mixed iris. These three broad categories represent different modes of human adaptation, and each embodies its own unique wisdom and sets the rules for its own methods of attempting to bring an individual back to health. Constitution by color is considered to be 100% inherited, and once developed in very early childhood, it will not change during the course of a life.

Primary constitutional iris types

The three primary constitutional iris types (see Figure 3.1):

1. Blue or blue-gray iris: lymphatic constitution
2. Dark brown iris: hematogenic constitution
3. Brown-green, brown-gray, hazel iris: mixed biliary constitution

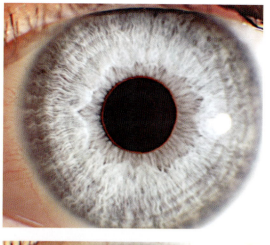

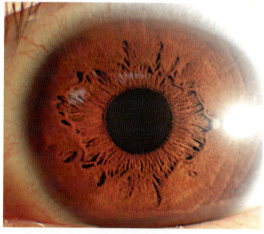

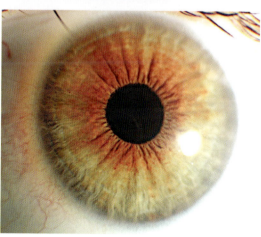

FIGURE 3.1

The three basic iris color types:
blue/blue-gray (top), pure dark brown (middle), and mixed/hazel (bottom).

These are very big categories, spread among the estimated 8 billion human inhabitants of the earth (at the time of writing). They are to be considered predominantly as adaptations to climatic conditions; however, in considering the different types, bear in mind that we all are basically constructed in the same way. The differentiation in eye color places us in certain physiologically behavioral modes, but the same concerns of metabolic balance through nutrition, detoxification, and harmonious hormonal and nerve impulses are present in us all.

THE BLUE/BLUE-GRAY IRIS

A blue or gray eye has no pigmentation except that reflected from the dark blue underlying layer of the stroma. If you look closely at a blue eye, it is hard to find any blue color. This type is known as the lymphatic constitution (Figure 3.2).

The fibers of the blue iris appear as whitish or gray. If the fibers are not very dense, the spaces between them may appear darker and bluer; dense, fine iris fibers will give a pale blue appearance, as they reflect more white light. Frequently there will be other bright white signs in these types, such as the ANW, or signs in the periphery of the iris known as tophi (Figure 3.3). (See "The Lymph Rosary," Chapter 5.)

Other colors, usually present in extremely small deposits and invisible to the naked eye, may sometimes be found in this type. (For a discussion of these additional signs and markings, see Chapter 7.)

The lymphatic constitution

If your eyes are purely or largely blue, ask yourself whether you have ever suffered from recurrent episodes of colds and sore throats, tonsillitis, excessive mucus, glandular swellings, hay fever, eczema, cystitis, irritable bowel syndrome, fever, or, later in life, rheumatic or arthritic pain.

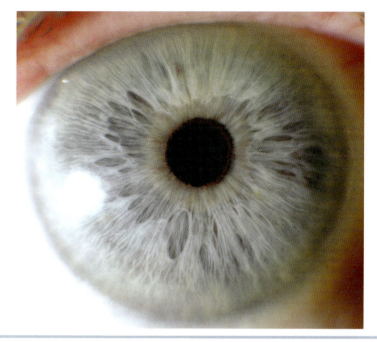

FIGURE 3.2

Blue/blue-gray iris: lymphatic type.

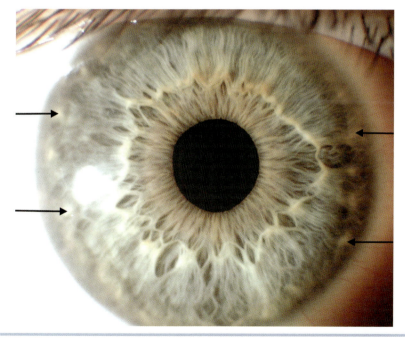

FIGURE 3.3

Lymphatic iris showing the presence of a lymph rosary.

The key element in all these complaints is *reactivity,* and the key physiological characteristic of this type is the ability to produce fast reactions to possible threats. This is considered to be a function of the origin of the blue-eyed type in colder Northern climes, where winters are often long and hard and there is sometimes limited sunlight or warmth from which energy may be derived.

Typical health concerns arise as a result of reactive inflammation in a tissue or organ. If something is irritating the tissues, the body will try to fight it. For example, when you catch a cold, the resulting inflammation is the body's attempt to fight the virus, or whatever influence it experiences as an irritant.

The term *lymphatic* refers to the system of the body that is concerned with the recycling of body fluids and the circulation of immune capacity. By recycling fluids, we keep the tissues of the body clean and unencumbered by waste products and toxins. Lymph, the fluid circulated in the lymphatic system, is clear plasma similar to blood, except that it contains only white blood cells, the job of which is to scavenge for and remove debris and to identify and kill anything that may be a threat to the system. In addition to drainage of the tissues, the lymph gland is an active component of our immune system. This is why the predominant physiological concerns of the lymphatic constitutional type are *elimination, detoxification,* and *immunity.*

Derivation of constitution

The blue-eyed type evolved in a cool climate (the Northern hemisphere), where generating and conserving heat was a primary need. However, generating and conserving heat also potentially leads to the increased generation and retention of waste products, which can provoke irritation and inflammation. The volume and kind of foods—particularly fats and carbohydrates—that blue-eyed types need to eat in order to generate warmth result in larger quantities of waste being produced.

Moreover, in order to preserve warmth, the skin and peripheral circulation need to be "closed down" against the cold. Normally the skin is an important organ of elimination through perspiration

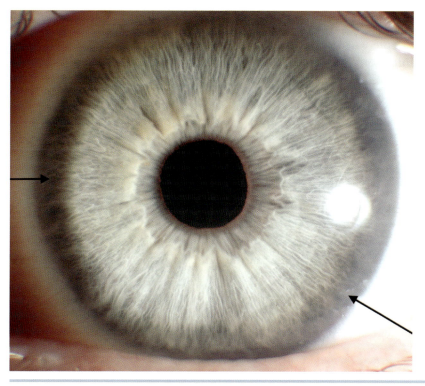

FIGURE 3.4

Lymphatic iris showing presence of the dark outer band or scurf rim.

and continuous respiration—releasing uric acid, carbon dioxide, and other metabolic wastes. If the skin is closed down, it is less able to carry out these functions. It is also inhibited in other jobs, such as shedding dead cells and collecting wastes for internal drainage in the "lymph zone," in the subcutaneous layers. In the iris this often appears as a dark outer band, known as a *scurf rim* (see also Chapter 7). (See Figure 3.4.)

Blue-eyed people, therefore, have a greater need for their bodies to react so that irritants are brought to their attention quickly. Reactivity is seen in the iris by the presence of whiteness. The degree of whiteness can vary considerably and indicates the degree of reactivity. You may notice, for example, that some fibers stand out particularly, or may appear in clusters: these indicate anatomical areas of high immune reactivity.

Common conditions

People with a lymphatic constitution have a tendency toward focal infections, fever, and inflammation. Blue-eyed children suffer from runny noses, sore throats, ear infections, and tonsillitis. They also may fall prey to eczema, hay fever, and other allergic conditions, which can often be traced to an excess of dairy produce and other mucus-forming and clogging foods in the diet, together with a weakening of the liver, kidneys, and skin in their detoxifying functions.

Irritable bowel syndrome (IBS) is also more common in people with blue irides due to this type's tendency to greater reactivity. IBS is an umbrella term that covers a range of possible symptoms but is frequently connected with food allergies and intolerances, disruption of the microbiome, and stress. Again, it is an inbuilt tendency to resort to inflammation and immune reactivity in order to address a problem.

IBS, along with other examples of reactivity, may also be driven by digestive insufficiency. The failure to break foods down properly has two downline consequences: malabsorption, where the nutrients contained in foods are not made available to us, thus depriving us of essential nutrition; and autointoxication, where the partially digested food molecules, particularly proteins, are regarded as toxic by your immune system, which then sets up a reactive process to try to neutralize the threat.

Accordingly, attention to digestive health is important. People with a lymphatic constitution tend toward being cold and damp, especially if out of balance or when health is compromised. *Damp*, in traditional medicine, is akin to stagnation and congestion, and *cold* is akin to lack of vitality and the ability to defend oneself. Hence over time we may also find that the natural reactivity with which these types are supplied starts to falter and wane, leaving the individual chronically undefended and struggling to find the energy to react to anything. One way of counteracting this is to reignite the "fire" of digestion—there are some great herbal suggestions for this below.

Detoxification, not suppression

In terms of terrain theory (see Chapter 1), we would always say that tissue cleanliness and vitality is the determining factor in our level of resistance, not the specific pathogen being highlighted (the cold "virus," etc.). High reactivity also implies high vitality, turning some of our cherished health notions on their heads. Most people would not consider the activity of the immune system in giving you a "cold" to be healthy, and yet, seen correctly, this is exactly the case. The immune reactivity is directed specifically at the elimination of irritants and of accumulations of waste products that may be undermining health, and there are ways to deal with this situation that do not involve suppressing it with pharmaceutical medications, but which assist and support the body's natural processes.

The habitual and typical response in our culture is to resort to the use of antibiotics to kill bacteria, painkillers and steroids to suppress inflammation, antihistamines to suppress an allergic response, or even the removal of "offending" body parts, such as the tonsils. This ultimately weakens the body and renders it less able to address its own problems. Unable to fight for itself, its immunity is compromised, while the toxic load continues to increase. The problems may disappear temporarily, only to return later as more serious, chronic complaints. The constant low-grade inflammation that then develops becomes destructive, leading to degeneration of body tissues and, in particular, diseases such as arthritis and rheumatism.

A more effective approach is to attempt to reduce the toxic load on the system by promoting natural detoxification and eliminating unhelpful foods from your diet.

The rheumatic type

A subgroup of pale blue-eyed individuals, the rheumatic type, typically display exaggerated defensive reactions, although they generally have strong constitutions and do not fall ill often. If they do become ill, this often takes the form of high, short-lived fevers, and they recover quickly. Their emotional reactions are similar: they may appear extreme at the time, but outbursts are infrequent and subside quickly. The irides of people of this type are characterized by a general whiteness of all the iris fibers (signifying reactivity), creating the visual impression of a very pale blue eye (Figure 3.5).

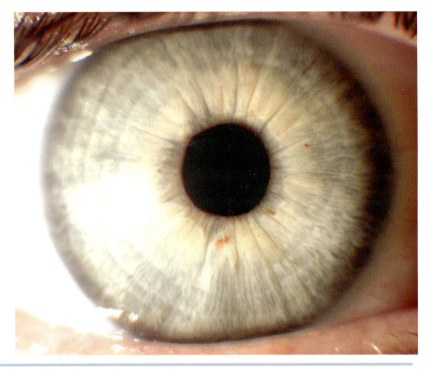

FIGURE 3.5

Lymphatic iris, rheumatic subtype.

Living with a lymphatic constitution

Tendencies of the blue iris type

▷ naturally adapted to a cooler climate;

▷ prone to disturbances of the lymphatic system, the body's drainage network;

▷ irritability of the mucous membranes, especially the upper respiratory tract, but also the gastrointestinal and urinary tracts and the skin;

▷ raised acid levels, disturbances of kidney function;

▷ rheumatic and allergic reactions;

▷ easy onset of fever.

There are a number of factors within your control that can help you avoid the problems to which you are prone. Among the most important of these are the foods that you eat and the supplements you take and certain specific activities that will contribute to wellbeing.

Dietary needs

Water: Making up more than 70% of your body's composition, water is required for flushing and regenerating body fluids, and for elimination and detoxification. The average person needs about two liters daily; those above average in height and weight may need more.

Fresh fruit and vegetables: These contain high levels both of water and of vitamins, minerals, antioxidants, and other micronutrients, which are essential for the maintenance of a healthy immune system. Fruit and vegetables—organic if possible—should constitute 60% of your diet, and up to 80% in warm weather. If you have a strong digestive system, eat as much raw food as possible, but if your digestion is below par, try gently steaming your vegetables, or taking warming soups and broths, particularly in winter, to assist digestion.

Oils and fats: These are important for generating warmth, especially in winter. Linseed, hempseed, and olive are largely monounsaturated and contain a good selection of essential fatty acids (EFAs). Excellent blends of nutritional oils are available in health food shops. Remember, the only "bad fats" are the highly heated fats the chemical structure of which has been changed—so-called "trans fats." Saturated fats (present in high amounts in coconut oil, palm oil) are fine for cooking with because they are inherently chemically stable. Unsaturated fats—e.g., virgin cold-pressed olive oil—relatively unstable and prone to oxidation, should always be used cold.

Foods to be avoided

Unfortunately, there are a large number of items that can interfere with the healthy maintenance of your immune system, including acid-producing and mucus-forming foods.

Dairy products: Milk, cheese, and cream, which are saturated fats, are mucus-forming and are frequently involved in disorders of the skin and mucous membranes, such as phlegm, eczema, hay fever, IBS, and asthma. If you do eat dairy, keep it to a minimum, and try to find raw or unpasteurized sources, where the enzyme content has not been destroyed.

Sugar and refined carbohydrates: It is now well publicized that these foods are highly detrimental to health, putting pressure on blood sugar regulation by contributing to insulin resistance, increasing levels of acidic byproducts that have to be handled by the detoxifying and eliminative mechanisms, and giving rise to free radicals, causing oxidative damage to cells. While a little can be tolerated in a healthy system, these highly "proinflammatory" foods are best avoided in ill health, especially if you are suffering from any chronic inflammatory complaint.

Processed food, and food additives: Processed food is not really food at all, having been created in a lab somewhere and rolled out to supermarkets for a profit. It is usually indigestible and creates waste products that the body's systems are ill equipped to handle. A well-known example is margarine—sold to the population in the 1950s as a miracle replacement for evil cholesterol-promoting dairy butter—but there are a thousand and one other examples on our supermarket shelves today.

Animal protein and fat: While animal protein and fat can be helpful for some, it is important to advise that such foods are not universally well digested and processed and can yield high levels of toxic byproducts. They will tend to slow down bowel motility and create congestion and autointoxication, whereby toxins are reabsorbed into the bloodstream. This applies particularly to hormonal problems in women: for example, when excess estrogen is broken down in the liver, the products are sent into the digestive tract for elimination, via bile secretion. There, in the presence of an enzyme called beta-glucuronidase, which tends to be high in meat-eating individuals, they may be restored to their original state and thus survive to get back into the blood stream and continue to disrupt the menstrual cycle. Eat animal protein and fat very moderately, if at all, and if you do eat meat, try to avoid red meat and pork.

Coffee, tea, alcohol, and carbonated or sugary drinks: These products, which are generally acid-forming, lead to increased dehydration, and the caffeinated versions also overstimulate the SNS, upsetting the delicate balance of the ANS. Cut them out or reduce your intake.

A healthy lifestyle

Skin brushing: Detoxification through the skin is a special need for lymphatic people, who frequently need to activate their skin. Perform dry skin brushing once daily, before bathing or showering. Take a fairly stiff bristle brush and work from the extremities in toward the heart in small vigorous circles, covering the entire area of the skin. Finish with large clockwise circles over the abdomen, following the direction of peristaltic flow of the colon. (For more information on dry skin brushing, see Chapter 10.)

Exercise: There are a number of activities that can promote the movement of lymph throughout the body, including yoga, Tai Chi, Qi Gong, swimming, and deep breathing. Deep breathing is very effective, because the main lymphatic vessel is the thoracic duct, which passes directly through the diaphragm. As the diaphragm moves with each breath, the thoracic duct is massaged, thus drawing lymph through the entire system.

The yoga postures in the Sun Salutation are also effective. Performing just one round is an excellent way to stimulate lymph. Other yoga poses contract and stretch the muscles of the chest, arms, and shoulders, massaging the nearby lymph nodes and encouraging lymph flow through the area. Poses like Downward Dog work and stretch the chest, as do back bends.

Even a simple exercise, such as bending backward over a bolster and stretching your arm over your head, can be very effective at stimulating lymph flow.

Regular detoxification periods: Occasionally, give up all unhealthy food and beverages, and drink more pure water (I recommend distilled water, as it contains nothing but H_2O). Regular cleansing protocols for certain key organs, such as the liver and kidneys, are to be encouraged. Detoxify your system at least three times a year, especially when the seasons change. One week of detoxification three or four times a year can have long-term benefits for your health (see Chapter 10).

Hydrotherapy: Hot and cold water can be used to stimulate circulation and move blood (Chapter 10). Sauna and steam baths are also excellent, but don't forget to take the cold plunge between bouts in the hot rooms.

Herbal choices

Herbal choices are based on the kinds of problems that tend to afflict the type. They are not reserved exclusively for the lymphatic constitution, but they are well suited to addressing their typical health concerns. (For preparing medicinal herbal teas, see "Herbal Preparations", in Chapter 10.)

Elderflower, yarrow, and peppermint (equal parts):   These herbs are gently diaphoretic—they open up the pores of the skin, allowing perspiration. This blend is my favorite for the onset of colds and the 'flu. Make as big an infusion as you can, and just keep drinking it at the first sign of trouble. You will find that the "infection" lasts a fraction of the time that you usually spend feeling ill, and your health will be restored, often within a day or so, and without the tail-end of mucous and stuffiness. Add fresh root ginger to the mix for extra warmth and protection.

The "alteratives" (blood and lymph cleansers):   These herbs work via diverse routes, such as promoting detoxification and elimination via liver, kidneys, and lymph. Alteratives often also have digestion-enhancing effects—poorly functioning digestion is one of the biggest contributory factors to autotoxemia—and are also sometimes relaxants and antispasmodics, counteracting stress, which is another significant source of toxicity within our systems.

Alteratives include dandelion, burdock, nettle, barberry bark, cleavers, yarrow, plantain, and red clover. Some of these herbs are also "antirheumatics," reducing chronic inflammation not by acting to suppress it, but by removing the causes and triggers of such inflammation.

Echinacea: This well-known immune stimulant and protector is known in traditional herbal medicine as a "lymphatic alterative." In particular, it promotes *phagocytosis*—the production of large white blood cells whose job it is to engulf, neutralize, break down, and remove toxic debris from the system.

Adaptogens and tonics: These herbs have very general effects in promoting the health of the immune system, adrenals, nerves, hormones, and much more. They are useful in assisting the body to adapt to stress, and restoring vitality if run down and weakened. They include astragalus root, Siberian ginseng root, schisandra berry, and ashwagandha (*Withania*) root, among many others. Many of them also improve the function of mitochondria—the energy-producing engines of our cells.

Digestive tonics and "carminative" herbs: Warming, activating, and relaxing digestion, these herbs counteract toxic buildup by ensuring the complete breakdown and absorption of foods within the digestive tract. They include ginger, peppermint, spearmint, rosemary, fennel seed, angelica root, caraway, cinnamon, and cardamom. They can be taken as a digestive tea after a large meal, with the benefit of assisting the digestion to complete its task efficiently. These herbs are also warming and stimulating to the circulation, counteracting any tendency toward cold and damp.

Diagnostic questions
(these questions assess the level of risk of the lymphatic type)

▷ Did you experience frequent infections, or tonsillitis, as a child?

▷ How is your immunity now?

▷ Do you suffer from allergies?

▷ Do you tend to produce a lot of mucous, or phlegm?

▷ Have you ever had significant suppressive treatments for immune problems (e.g., antibiotics, antihistamines)?

Positive suggestions for the lymphatic type

▷ Your immune system is always doing the right thing—look after it, and it will look after you.

▷ Thank your symptoms for showing you the way to better health. (For the lymphatic type, see Figure 3.2 above.)

THE PURE DARK BROWN IRIS

The pure dark brown color may vary from one individual to another, and there may be areas of darker or lighter pigmentation in the same iris, but generally people of this type are noted for irides that are smooth, homogenous, and of a velvety texture. This type is known as the hematogenic constitution. (See Figure 3.6.)

The thick brown pigment found in this type is sometimes described as a "chromatophoric carpet": *chromatophore* is the name given to the cells that secrete this particular pigment. The fibers in this iris type are not visible, because they are completely obscured by the dense pigmentation, which penetrates all four layers of the stroma. It is therefore described as "total pigmentation," with all pigment-secreting cells "turned on," genetically speaking. In this regard it is interesting to note that there is no inherent anatomical difference between the blue iris and the dark brown iris, except for this hypersecretion of pigment. If you could remove this pigment, you would end up with a blue iris.

Sometimes, in order to distinguish between the pure dark

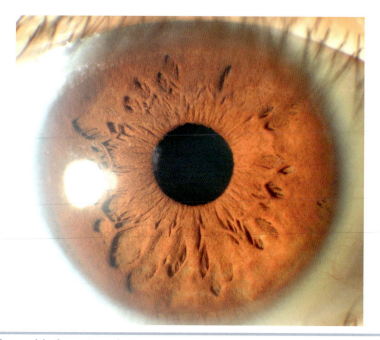

FIGURE 3.6

The pure dark brown iris: hematogenic type.

brown type iris and the lighter or more variegated types (see mixed iris, below), you will need to use magnification or photography, as the naked eye will not pick up the more minute variations in color that reveal a mixed-type iris. The pure dark brown, or hematogenic iris, is distinguished by the invisibility of iris fibers within the main body of the iris.

The hematogenic constitution

The pure, velvet-brown type iris is called the hematogenic type (from the Greek word *haem*, meaning blood). The key indications for people of this type involve blood composition (sugars, fats, minerals, electrolytes, and hormones) and blood dynamics (blood pressure and circulation).

This iris type's dense pigmentation makes it difficult to see the precise arrangement of the fibers, and iridologists often complain that hematogenic irides are somewhat difficult to read. In fact, there is usually plenty to see, but this depends on putting in sufficient practice and time looking for the relevant signs and indications. You will need a bright light, and good magnification or suitable photography, to examine pure brown irides.

Distinguishing between pure brown and mixed iris types

If you think you have pure brown eyes, check the color carefully—to the naked or unpracticed eye, dark mixed iris types may be difficult to distinguish from the pure brown iris. Here are some features in the iris that can help you determine whether you are actually a dark mixed iris type:

 ▷ Irides are mainly brown, but there is an edge of green around the periphery.
 ▷ Irides look brown, but on closer inspection there is blue or green visible beneath the superficial layer, where it is interrupted by a lacuna (a hole in the texture).
 ▷ Irides are mainly brown, but the individual fibers are visible through occasionally thin, cloudy, brown pigment.

If any of these descriptions match your irides, you may have a darker version of the *mixed iris type* rather than the pure brown type. (See Figure 3.7.)

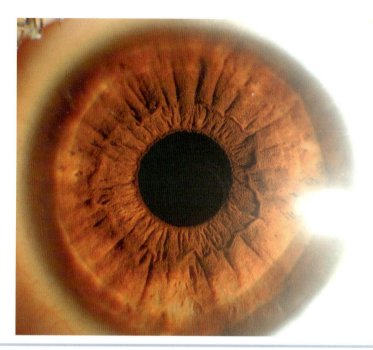

FIGURE 3.7

Very dark "mixed" iris: note the greenish patches in the lower sector.

Derivation of constitution

Pure brown eyes predominate among African and Asian people, which gives rise to the theory that this iris type evolved in a hotter climate, the pigmentation being a protective measure (see Chapter 2). That, however, is not to say that the type only occurs in this demographic. There are also fair-skinned people who have this iris type, and, by the same token, there are dark-skinned people with blue or pale irides. The rule in iridology is that it is the *iris*, not the skin or the nominal racial type, that determines the constitution. Thus a blue eye is a lymphatic type, no matter in whom it occurs, and a dark brown eye is a hematogenic type, no matter if the skin is not also dark.

People with pure dark brown irides probably account for more than 60% of the world's population, so it is perhaps surprising that not more has been written about identifying their unique characteristics. While a range of variations has been recognized and documented for lighter eye colors (see discussion of overlay types, in Chapter 5), only two or three subtypes are typically listed for the hematogenic iris. However, in practice, most of the variants noted in the lymphatic type can be found to some extent in the hematogenic type as well—you just need to know what to look for.

Common conditions

Pure brown-eyed people are physiologically generally less reactive. They do not tend to suffer from the inflammatory responses or early onset of complications affecting the mucous membranes, skin, and lymphatic tissue that characterize the blue-eyed person. Brown-eye disorders are usually characterized by a slow onset and gradual accumulation, leading to disturbance of normal function. The key word here is *compensation*: these systems will tolerate a buildup, up to a point, and one danger of this is that problems build up unnoticed: the symptoms that might act as warnings are generally absent, or subtle enough not to be picked up in everyday life.

Processes tend to be more hidden; reaction and inflammation are slower to appear. That is why major diseases found in pure brown-eyed people tend to surface later in life and be relatively serious, being the long-term results of a gradual progression of metabolic disturbances. It is, therefore, important to catch and treat symptoms when they arise.

If a hematogenic person is found to display frequent lymphatic-type symptoms, such as allergic reactions and infective crises, which in a blue-eyed person might be considered "normal," this would suggest that the underlying disorder has progressed to a more serious level. Fever, for example, is generally a more serious problem for hematogenic constitutions.

Detoxification, therefore, is just as important to the hematogenic type as to the lymphatic. Accumulations may build up undetected for years, and their influence may be more destructive for not having been dealt with sooner. Once accumulation has reached unsupportable levels, the descent into "pathology" can be swift.

Examples of this are frequently encountered of this type: "My blood pressure was always low, then in mid-life it suddenly went up massively"; "I used to experience bouts of low blood sugar (hypoglycemia), but then, when I was in my 40s, I was unexpectedly diagnosed with Type 2 diabetes."

Blood-related disorders

Statistically, people with pure dark brown irides are known to have an above-average tendency toward diabetes, high blood fats (including cholesterol), and other rarer and more specific disturbances of blood composition, such as various types of anemia. However, these are usually the full-blown end results of a lifetime spent in ignorance of this particular constitution and its needs. Such blood-related disorders may include:

Poor circulation: Blood tends to be thicker in people of the hematogenic type, and many brown-eyed people living in colder climes will suffer from circulatory problems: capillaries contract in cold weather, and the thicker blood cannot penetrate the narrow peripheral vessels. The result is extreme cold experienced in hands and feet. (See also below, "Anemia, blood deficiency, and blood stagnation.")

Blood sugar issues: This is a big concern for hematogenic types, and many exhibit already in childhood and youth the early signs of Type 2 diabetes, including strong cravings for sweet foods and feeling faint, nauseous, or irritable when hungry ("hangry"!).

It should be remembered, however, that hypoglycemia (low blood sugar), which produces these symptoms, is the other side of the diabetes coin and is also an indicator of digestive insufficiency, whereby energy and vitality are not being serviced adequately by digestion, and so the body craves easy energy in the form of sugars.

Sugar is easily absorbed with a minimum of digestive effort, and so serves to lift energy levels fast and effectively—but with a price to pay. Simple sugar is "fast-burn" energy, lifting levels quickly, but dropping them just as fast, resulting in further craving. Additionally, over time, the acidic metabolic residues of excess sugar consumption lead to increased oxidative damage and subsequent inflammation (leading to, among other conditions, cholesterol deposits in the arteries—another big risk factor of the type); continual "spiking" of insulin results in insulin resistance and eventually diabetes; and the body is starved of essential nutrients from wholesome foods, which are being replaced by easy options.

High cholesterol and risk of atherosclerosis: Narrowing of the arteries due to cholesterol buildup is attributed to high levels in the blood; however, cholesterol plaquing in the arteries is, in fact, driven by inflammation and also involves other mineral substances that are precipitated "out of solution" to effect temporary repairs to the inner arterial surfaces. The hematogenic iris type is more than usually prone to develop the so-called cholesterol ring, which may appear as a whitish ring around the outer circle of the iris. (For a full discussion, see Chapter 5.)

High blood pressure: Although all types may develop this condi-tion—as, indeed, the cholesterol situation too—it is especially common in the hematogenic type, where, as noted above, it can occur quite quickly and with little notice. Two common causes may be considered: stress, and the effects of stress; and *resistance* caused by accumulation and toxemia, whereby the body tries to overcome the resistance by forcing the pressure up in order to get much-needed nutrients and oxygen to areas where they are needed.

Anemia, blood deficiency, and blood stagnation: There are some types of anemia that are predominantly found in individuals with this iris type, including sickle cell anemia and thalassemia. These conditions are caused by abnormalities of red blood cells, such that they cannot carry oxygen effectively to the tissues of the body.

However, this type is also predisposed to anemia through iron deficiency, and through general blood deficiency. "Blood deficiency" is a term used in traditional medicine—for example, Chinese medicine—to describe a condition in which blood is poorly nourished and poorly oxygenated and thus cannot supply tissue with adequate nutrients, resulting in a generally devitalized state. (For a discussion of the "anemia ring," frequently found in this type, see Chapter 7.)

Blood deficiency may also be found in conjunction with *blood stagnation*—another term in traditional medicine—which refers to thickening and sluggishness of the blood and circulation. It is associated microscopically with the phenomenon of "aggluti-nation," where red blood cells are found to be sticking to one another; this is also known as *erythrocyte clumping* (erythrocyte = red blood cell).

Hormones: Hormones are blood-borne, and they depend on healthy blood and healthy circulation for correct function. All hormonal pathways and functions are potentially affected, but the reproductive hormones, especially in women, are a particular focus for attention.

Clots, stones, and lumps: A general tendency toward accumulation and excess means hematogenic women may experience heavy menstruation, with dark, clotted menstrual blood. Also common in both sexes are hard, crystalline deposits, such as kidney stones and gallstones (often associated with high cholesterol), and lumps, cysts, and tumors of all kinds.

Tumors, considered to be a possibly life-threatening occurrence, potentially represent an attempt to isolate toxic or otherwise compromising material. Hard deposits and formations are accumulations of matter that have not been resolved through normal channels of detoxification and elimination and must be kept out of the way of the body's normal processes.

Stress and anxiety: The hematogenic constitution has been shown to be especially subject to higher levels of *emotional* responsiveness or reactivity.[2] This trait may, to some extent, be regarded as an emotional correlate to the storage of extraneous matter that the body has not been able to eliminate. It may also have to do with the fact that many individuals with this constitution also have a self-protective disposition (Figure 3.8), which is itself predisposed to anxiety and neuromuscular tension (see Chapter 4).

Living with a hematogenic constitution

Tendencies of the pure dark brown iris type

> natural adaptation to a warm or hot climate;

> disturbances of blood composition: thick blood, high blood fats, blood sugar abnormalities, mineral deficiencies;

> disturbances of hormone activity (hormones are transported by the blood);

> tendency to formation of stones and other accumulations;

> hidden or "subacute" disease processes;

> low reactivity, a more serious condition when fever does occur.

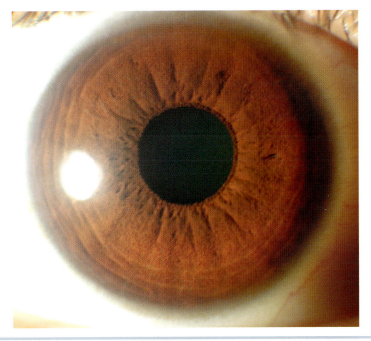

FIGURE 3.8

Hematogenic iris with self-protective disposition.

There are a number of factors within your control that can help you avoid the problems to which you are prone. Among the most important of these are the foods that you eat and the supplements you take, as well as certain specific activities that will contribute to wellbeing.

Dietary needs

Foods that nourish and cleanse the blood are the most important for this type (see below), and there is also a need for blood-moving spices—several of these can be found below in the herbal section.

If a hematogenic person was born in and has lived in a hot country and then moves to a colder country, he or she should adhere as closely as possible to the diet of their country of origin. Diets in hot countries often involve the use of peppery spices, which stimulate digestion and circulation. Adopting the indigenous dietary habits of a colder country, which include more fat, sugar, and carbohydrate, will aggravate the typical hematogenic constitutional sensitivities.

Blood-builders: Eat plenty of fresh fruit and vegetables, particularly blood-building dark-green leafy vegetables and red, purple, and black fruits (e.g., berries), for minerals (especially iron), antioxidants, and trace elements. Drink lots of freshly pressed juices and smoothies, which are excellent food supplementation. The nutrition in juices is instantly available and wholly absorbable as all the "packaging" cellulose is removed. The so-called superfoods can also be used to similar effect (see Chapter 10).

Wholegrains: Eat brown or whole-grain products, such as pasta, bread, and rice, as opposed to denatured "white carbs"—the parts of the grain that are stripped away in processing contain the natural oils, minerals, and vitamins that make them worth consuming in the first place.

Foods to be avoided

Sugar and refined carbohydrates: To prevent or delay the onset of blood sugar disturbances and diabetes, keep high-glycemic foods to a minimum. These foods are also highly proinflammatory and mucus-forming, and they contribute heavily to overloaded and undernourished blood.

Saturated fats and cholesterol: While cholesterol itself is not necessarily the medical bugaboo it has been made out to be, it is also true that rich, fat-laden foods will exacerbate the tendencies of the type, thickening blood and contributing to stagnation and congestion.

Caffeine and other stimulants: Avoid the hyperstimulation of caffeine, alcohol, and other stimulating substances, which contribute to stress and tension, as well as increasing acidic residues.

A healthy lifestyle

Stress management: Stress demands huge amounts of energy and nutritional power. Those with a hematogenic constitution may not be aware of its adverse effects until these are serious. Learn to relax (see Chapter 10). Stress is a key factor in the onset of high cholesterol levels and high blood pressure.

Keep warm: Hematogenic types living in cold climates will tend to have difficulty keeping circulation active and vital. Try visiting a spa and perform regular hydrotherapy work to stimulate and revitalize circulation.

Exercise: Cardiovascular exercise, in particular, will maintain the health of the heart and circulatory vessels. Keep active, and remember that your body needs to move. Enjoy physical activity and let it take you out of repetitive, anxiety-producing thought patterns.

Regular detoxification: Detox is a requirement for all types, but it may have different focuses for different types. In the hematogenic type, the target is blood composition, so we need to be thinking of the ways in which the body maintains blood in a healthy state. All avenues of elimination should be targeted regularly, but especially the liver (see Chapter 10).

Herbal choices

Herbal choices are based on the kinds of problems that tend to afflict the type. They are not reserved exclusively for the hematogenic constitution, but they are well suited to addressing their typical health concerns. (For instructions on preparing medicinal herbs, see "Herbal Preparations", in Chapter 10.)

Blood-movers and circulatory stimulants: To overcome the tendency to sluggish circulation, use hot spices, such as cayenne, ginger, garlic, and horseradish. These can be used as strong herbal extracts or simply as spices in food. Milder spices, such as cinnamon, cardamom, and fennel, are also useful; these spices are also digestive stimulants. Garlic and cayenne are also helpful in maintaining clear arterial passages and reducing cholesterol and blood pressure.

Blood-nourishing herbs: These herbs fortify deficient blood. They include Dong Quai (Chinese angelica), one of the most useful blood nourishers and blood-movers and a powerful hormonal remedy for women, also working via the liver to ensure the correct metabolization of hormones. Also consider nettle (high in iron and other minerals), and *Angelica archangelica* (European angelica), a digestive stimulant that is also known to enhance the absorption of iron. Under this category also appear bone-marrow tonics (bone marrow is the production site for blood cells)—an excellent combination is astragalus root and yellow dock root, which can be taken either as a tincture or as a decoction (see Chapter 10).

Digestive stimulants and cholagogues: Cholagogues stimulate the production of bile, specifically, and are thereby useful for the breakdown of fats in the digestive system; they specifically help to balance and metabolize cholesterol. They include artichoke leaf, barberry bark, dandelion root and leaf, and burdock root. They generally have a very bitter taste, and, appropriately, they are also good for counteracting cravings for sweet foods; they are hence are protective against diabetes.

Alteratives: The qualities of alterative herbs have been discussed in the section on the lymphatic constitution. It is highly important for the hematogenic constitution not to allow too much accumulation of deleterious substances, so regular detoxification is part of the preventive strategy. For this type, the deep-cleansing "woody" alteratives—roots and root barks—are particularly sought after; they include dandelion, barberry root bark, and burdock root. (These herbs are all, also, cholagogues.)

One of the most useful alteratives for general purposes, however, is red clover flower. This herb gently cleanses and restores blood, while also relaxing the system; it is a powerful guard against accumulations leading to hard deposits and tumors. Best taken as a refreshing, fragrant herbal tea.

Heart- and circulation-supporting: Motherwort, hawthorn, lime flowers, and wild oat tinctures relax and calm; they also help to balance cholesterol and lower blood pressure.

Diagnostic questions
(these questions assess the level of risk of the hematogenic type)

▷ Do you crave sweet foods or carbohydrates?

▷ Do you have a family history of blood sugar issues, including Type 2 diabetes?

▷ Do you have a family history of high cholesterol or cardiovascular disease, including high blood pressure?

▷ Have you ever been diagnosed with anemia?

▷ Do you suffer with cold extremities or sluggish circulation?

Positive suggestions for the hematogenic type:

▷ You have a strong ability to withstand the stresses and strains of life.

▷ Your blood is your strength: keep it clean and free-flowing. (See Figure 3.9.)

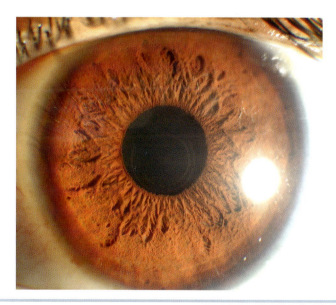

FIGURE 3.9

A further example of a hematogenic iris.

THE MIXED (LIGHT BROWN OR HAZEL) IRIS

Mixed irides, which include green or hazel eyes, are very varied in the distribution and intensity of pigment. They may be quite dark, so that it is difficult to distinguish them from the pure dark brown iris type, or quite pale, as in the green iris type. This type is known as the *mixed biliary constitution.* (See Figure 3.10.)

Generally, pigment is denser over the central region of the iris, around the pupil, and there may be some significant fading of this toward the edges of the iris, so that the underlying blue or gray can be seen. The mixed iris type is also distinguishable by the visibility of at least some of the individual iris fibers, usually toward the edge, where the pigment becomes thinner. There will often be pigment patches or spots in the outer zone.

Green eyes are not actually green. The basic color of the iris is either blue or gray, and over this appears either a thin layer of yellow or light brown pigment, or else specific, quite sharply defined, patches of color—usually yellow or brown. The eye of the observer puts this together and sees green (see Figure 3.11.)

The mixed biliary constitution

The full name of this type is *mixed biliary.* The biliary tract refers specifically to liver and gallbladder; however, for iridological purposes we include the stomach and the pancreas, as well as the entire digestive tract. An important key phrase is *enzyme provision*: a typical shortfall in this is often responsible for the common complaints of the type.

Relevant questions to ask might include: do you suffer with any digestive complaints (e.g., indigestion, gastroesophageal reflux, bloating, flatulence, constipation, or diarrhea)? However, do not be put off if the person responds that, on the contrary, their digestion is near perfect, and they have no issues. Many a mixed type has already learned their lesson in that regard and has made the appropriate changes to their diet and their eating habits, such that they no longer suffer with such symptoms.

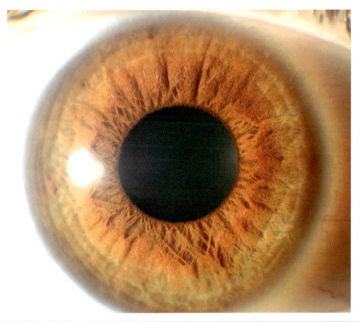

FIGURE 3.10

Brown-gray or hazel iris: mixed biliary type.

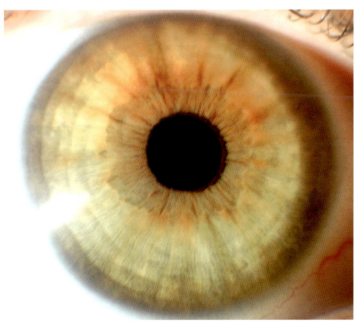

FIGURE 3.11

Light mixed biliary type showing greenish hue.

This neatly illustrates a crucial factor in iridology: that there is no such thing as a "good" or "bad" iris constitution—it all depends on how you live with what you've got.

Derivation of constitution

The mixed iris type represents two different sources of genetic information and bears characteristics of both, to varying degrees. Darker and denser pigmentation pushes the constitution toward the hematogenic iris type, and greener irides may lean toward lymphatic concerns. Energetically, people of the mixed iris type embody a conflict between the slower, more measured process of the hematogenic person and the often intemperate reactivity of the lymphatic person. However, if the individual is in balance, then the mixed iris type has the best of both worlds in terms of adaptation.

Whether someone is a dark mixed or hematogenic type may be less significant than supposed, as the implications are similar for the two. In the same way, many blue irides have patches of yellow, orange, or brown, placing them between a light mixed type and lymphatic type. Where pigment is a feature, it must enter the interpretation and will inevitably modify the picture and recommendations for the types.

Common conditions

Pigment in the mixed iris type is thicker over the central portion of the iris, and this is where iridology charts place the reflex to the gastrointestinal tract, meaning that the inherent health sensitivities of the mixed type are specifically digestive. The effect of pigment is always to slow things down, and mixed-type people have a particular tendency toward a sluggish digestion. There may be a reduced supply of digestive enzymes from the liver, gallbladder, and pancreas, resulting in discomfort, particularly after large, heavy meals or when trying to digest too many food types at once. Bloating, belching, and flatulence are common, as is also a tendency to constipation.

Indigestion, epigastric bloating, and gastroesophageal reflux disease: In taking a case, I am always careful to ask not just *if* a person experiences bloating, but *when* this tends to happen. Epigastric bloating suggests that food is not being processed appropriately in the stomach itself; this starts soon after beginning to eat a meal—even before the meal is finished. Stomach acid, specifically, will be found to be low, and the phenomenon of "delayed gastric emptying" applies.

Gastroesophageal reflux disease (GERD)—also known as "acid reflux"—is often erroneously treated by the pharmaceutical and medical professions with the use of "antacids" and drugs that suppress the production of acids in the system, such as the "PPIs" (proton pump inhibitors). If the problem is caused by not having enough stomach acid in the first place, how is it going to be solved by suppressing what minimal production there is? Sure enough, the symptom is suppressed: with no acid to burn the interior surfaces of the lower esophagus, the pain disappears. But digestion and absorption are impaired, and the overall health of the digestive tract suffers accordingly.

Upward regurgitation of stomach contents is caused by delayed gastric emptying and by the weakness of the lower esophageal sphincter (LOS). There is a natural reflex mechanism whereby the production of stomach acid automatically tightens the LOS, thus preventing upward leakage. Insufficient gastric acid, therefore, contributes to reflux; also, the longer the contents remain in the stomach, the more chance of them being upwardly displaced into the esophagus—as, for example, if you move about too much, or lie down, having eaten too much too late in the evening.

The natural and herbal response to this situation is described below, under "Herbal Choices".

Dysbiosis: If the natural population of gut bacteria has become disturbed, partly due to dietary factors, but also because of insufficient gastrointestinal immunity and an inability to prevent less friendly organisms from causing disruption, this may lead to dysbiosis. A well-cited example of this is *candidosis*: infestation with the *Candida albicans* fungus that is also the cause of thrush. However, in line with terrain theory, remember that it is never the organism that is to blame, but a disturbed environment in which the health-producing elements are unable to prevail.

Leaky gut syndrome: Everything that happens in the upper section of the digestive tract—starting with the mouth and including the stomach and the duodenum, where food is combined with juices from the liver/gallbladder and the pancreas—is vital in determining the health status of the lower digestive tract. Failure to digest properly in the upper portion will lead to potentially toxic substances—especially partly digested proteins—entering the lower regions, the small and large intestines, resulting in disturbance of the microbiome (natural gut bacteria), undermining gastrointestinal immunity and even permitting toxins to enter the bloodstream and contributing to inflammatory processes elsewhere in the body.

It is also as well to remember that poor digestion may not always exhibit direct symptoms. Failure to break foods down and absorb them sufficiently can lead to metabolic deficiencies, for example, in the endocrine system (the pituitary, thyroid, and adrenal glands), in the endocrine function of the pancreas, and even in the testes/ovaries, affecting reproductive capacity. These types of concerns are also shared with hematogenic-type people.

Blood sugar irregularities: The flip side of poorly functioning digestion is disturbance of blood sugar regulation, as has already been discussed. When experiencing difficulty in generating sufficient energy from healthier foods, the body looks for easy options in simple sugars and carbohydrates, which spike insulin and put pressure on the pancreas. Diabetes can be the chronic result.

Constipation and diarrhea: Problems with bowel motility are frequently encountered with the mixed biliary type. This will most often be bowel sluggishness—constipation—at least partly due to insufficiency of bile secretion. Bile is a natural laxative, and I have had many a mixed type in my clinic presenting with constipation; taking herbal "bitters" before each meal has pretty much solved their problem (see the herbal section below).

In the case of diarrhea, this is usually to be found in the lighter or paler types, where the natural reactivity of the lymphatic constitution may be putting in an appearance. Again, however, in addition to poor food choices and potential sensitivities, it is the failure to process foods adequately in the upper digestive tract that is often the cause of this symptom. However, diarrhea is also associated with a disturbed microbiome, so attention to this factor is a must.

Generation of toxins and "damp":   In traditional medicine terms, a major cause of toxin accumulation, dampness, and "phlegm" is a poorly functioning digestion. This will potentially affect all types, not just the mixed, but the mixed may be more prone due to the particularities of their constitution. (See the discussion of damp in the section above on the lymphatic constitution.)

The "urinary" type

The lighter mixed coloration is sometimes called the *urinary type,* because the urinary system may be a particular concern of the greener types. People of this type share more of the lymphatic type's concerns about detoxification and elimination, due to a greater percentage of the underlying blue color showing through in the iris. There may also be a hyperacidic overlay (see Chapter 5). There can be a tendency for sluggish conditions in the digestive tract to affect the kidneys, through the creation of toxins that slow down or impair kidney function. (See Figure 3.12.)

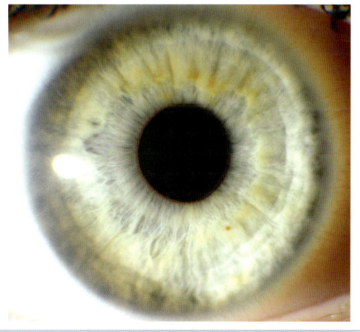

FIGURE 3.12

Very light mixed iris: urinary type.

Living with a mixed constitution

There are a number of factors within your control that can help you avoid the problems to which your iris type is prone. Among the most important of these are the foods you eat and the supplements you take, as well as certain specific activities that will contribute to wellbeing. Make sure you also check the recommendations for the pure brown-eyed and blue-eyed types, which also may be relevant to you.

Tendencies of the mixed iris type

Genetically a mix of the two opposite constitutions—blue and dark brown—and potentially exhibiting symptoms consistent with either, depending on the degree of pigmentation.

> disturbance of digestive function on all levels, resulting from sluggish or insufficient secretion of digestive fluids and enzymes;

> consequences of malabsorption, including fatigue and nutritional deficiency;

> dysbiosis and disorders of gastrointestinal immunity, including leaky gut syndrome;

> blood sugar irregularities and diabetes;

> constipation and/or diarrhea.

Dietary needs

Mealtime hygiene: It may be said, with considerable justification, that it is as important for this type to pay attention to *how* they eat, as it is to *what* they eat. The rules of "mealtime hygiene" will enable the optimal use of the digestive capacity, whatever that is, and are as follows (these rules may be applied to *everyone*, with benefits galore!)

Rules of mealtime hygiene

> Always eat in a calm, relaxed atmosphere, and **never** when upset, busy, or stressed out. To digest properly, your parasympathetic nervous system ("rest and digest") needs to be engaged. If you are in sympathetic mode ("fight or flight"), you will

not be able to digest efficiently, if at all. There is a reason why in some countries lunch (the main meal) is taken very seriously and time is allowed for a "siesta" afterwards, to ensure complete digestion.

▷ Chew all foods thoroughly. Digestion begins in the mouth, where carbohydrates, in particular, are predigested with salivary amylase. Breaking foods down into smaller particles is also crucial and eases the task of the stomach. Opinions vary as to how many times it is necessary to chew: between 20 times and 40 times. I go with 30, for good measure.

▷ Do not eat too many different food types in one sitting. To do so puts too much demand on an already suboptimal system. A worst-case scenario for many mixed types would be a five-course banquet: it is unlikely that they would make it to the end! Food-combining rules may be appropriate here.

▷ ***Do not overeat***: this cannot be overemphasized. Overeating is one of the biggest causes of inflammation—in fact, probably equal to or closely behind stress. There is a subtle signal that can be detected if one is eating with calm attention, which lets you know when your system has had enough. It owes this to a hormone released in the small intestine, called leptin, whose function is to inhibit hunger. It is rather subtle: if you are not paying attention, you will miss it, but it can be discerned with practice and is not to be overridden.

▷ Do not dilute digestive juices by drinking too much with meals. A little water to clear the palate is fine, but avoid washing food down with gallons of fluids.

▷ Conversely, however, drinking around half a pint of water 30 minutes before a meal can provide the liver and pancreas with sufficient fluid with which to manufacture the secretions we need for digestion.

▷ Do not eat too late at night; leave at least three hours between your last meal and retiring to bed. Once you are asleep, no digestion will take place—or, at least, it will take place very slowly. The optimal time for your main meal of the day is lunch-time, but this rarely suits our current cultural work patterns, so do what you can to eat early in the evening: 8 pm should be the cutoff point.

Soups, broths, and mild spices: In many traditions, digestion is likened to a fire. In cases of deficient digestion, it is necessary to not put the fire out, so cold and damp foods are not recommended, especially if symptoms are present. This includes raw foods, because digesting raw foods requires the digestion to be able to break down cellulose—a very tough constituent of plant foods—and without some help it is sometimes going to struggle with this. Applying heat (cooking—but not overcooking) is therefore recommended as a digestive aid: steam vegetables at least until comfortably crunchy (*al dente,* as the Italians might say). Warming soups and broths are ideal, together with mild spices such as fennel seed, cardamom pods, cinnamon bark, coriander seed, cumin seed, and so forth.

Bitter greens salads and other appetizers: A tossed green salad of rocket leaf, watercress, dandelion leaf, sorrel, and baby spinach, served with a splash of organic cold-pressed olive oil, has the effect of priming digestive fluids before the main event. The bitter taste is an automatic kick-start to digestion, so by the time the main course comes along, your stomach will be ready.

This is similar to the idea of *antipasti*: small servings of pickles, olives, and so forth as starters, the sour taste being stimulating to digestion.

Juices and smoothies: Although in some cases contraindicated due to being cold and damp, these preparations may relieve the load on digestive organs by supplying high-quality nutrition at low digestive cost, while assisting detoxification and immunity. The rule is, ensure all fruits and vegetables are juiced fresh prior to consumption, as opposed to being shop-bought or otherwise stored. This way the full enzyme content survives to assist the digestive processes. Juices and smoothies can be energetically "warmed up" by adding ginger, cayenne, or garlic. However, caution is necessary if you have any tendency toward diabetes, as the concentration of sugars and carbohydrates may spike insulin levels.

Foods to be avoided

Saturated fats and trans-fats: There is some controversy at the time of writing regarding the desirability or not of consuming saturated versus poly- and monounsaturated fats. I am not going to get into the pros and cons of this, save to suggest that if the secretion of bile from the liver is insufficient to needs, then any concentrated fat is going to prove difficult to digest. Therefore, I generally advise caution with full-fat dairy produce (especially bovine), meats such as beef, lamb, and pork, and baked goods— especially if prepared using refined flour and sugar. These may cause epigastric fullness and bloating and even nausea, and are best avoided if you have any digestive symptoms.

Refined carbohydrates: Enough has been said about the dangers of these for them to be contraindicated in any case of digestive deficiency.

A healthy lifestyle

Mealtime hygiene: This cannot be overstated, so I am saying it again: take your time over meals, do not overeat, and concentrate on enjoying the food. Eating in a hurry places stress upon constitutional sensitivities and will result in disturbances.

Enjoy yourself: Mixed types may have a need to become settled in the physical body, to accept it and find peace with it. The parasympathetic nerves regulate digestion, and these are also activated by recreation and relaxation.

Exercise: After eating, walking or light recreational exercise is beneficial for digestion. Many yoga positions assist the digestive organs; for example, inverted postures (shoulder stand, headstand) aid bowel function and relieve constipation; twists and forward bends massage the internal organs; and "nauli" (the contraction and isolation of abdominal muscles) provides strong stimulation of the digestive organs.

Herbal choices

Bitters, or bitter tonics: In herbal medicine, digestion-stimulating herbs, including gentian root, centaury herb, barberry bark, wormwood, and dandelion leaf are known as "bitter tonics": they act to stimulate digestive secretions across the board—in stomach, liver/gallbladder, and pancreas, but also starting in the mouth: observe for yourself the effect of taking something bitter on the tongue. Saliva is the second stage of digestion (the first being in the mind, at the smell, sight, or anticipation of food). Bitter herbs are also cholagogues, cooling and draining the liver, increasing the flow of bile, and thereby also helping to relieve constipation (bile is a natural laxative).

There are several interesting things about bitters that are deserving of attention. One is that they work by direct contact with bitter taste receptors on the tongue. They do not have to enter the stomach in order to stimulate digestion. This is called "neurogenic switching," or reflex action. Another highly intriguing fact is that, according to the Chinese *Yellow Emperor's Classic of Internal Medicine* (the *Huangdi Ne Ching*), the bitter flavor is said to enter, not the liver, not the stomach, but the *heart*! Modern research recently revealed that there are taste receptors sensitive specifically to bitters located in the inner walls of the human heart. Who knew? The ancient Chinese did, evidently!

Bitters are also employed in Western herbal medicine to treat hormonal, or endocrine, disturbances, especially blood sugar irregularities. Without good digestion, the building blocks of hormonal activity are lacking, so adequate provision of nutrients is very important to the hormonal system.

Carminatives: As also discussed in the lymphatic section, carminatives are warming and relaxing (antispasmodic) to the digestive system. Use peppermint, spearmint, rosemary, basil, oregano, and citrus peel to help relieve intestinal gas and spasm. These can also be combined with bitters to make a more well-rounded mix, with a pleasant-enough flavor. Some herbs—angelica, mugwort, and ginger, for example—are also regarded as "hot" or warming bitters.

Bitter tonic recipe:

You will need:

- *30% barberry bark*
- *15% fennel seed*
- *15% citrus peel*
- *15% peppermint leaf*
- *10% gentian root*
- *10% wormwood leaf*
- *5% ginger*

Combine tinctures of these herbs in the proportions indicated. Take 15 drops directly on the tongue, just before each meal.

Antispasmodics: In addition to the antispasmodic effects of the carminative herbs, smooth-muscle relaxant herbs, such as wild yam, cramp bark, and skullcap, can assist in cases of stress and tension held in the digestive tract. Remember the necessity to be calm and relaxed while eating.

Cathartics: Cascara bark, senna leaf or pod, and aloe gel will help move the bowels if the bitter/cholagogue approach does not work. It is important to work on the underlying cause of constipation, however, rather than relying on these very powerful laxatives. This may variously highlight food choices (too much meat, dairy, and refined carbohydrate), hydration levels (a common cause of constipation is dehydration), and tension affecting the gut (use antispasmodics).

Demulcent and mucilaginous herbs: These herbs generally have a content of mucilage—a slippery carbohydrate substance that acts to lubricate, soothe, and cool the internal surfaces of the gut—and are indicated for GERD, gastritis, types of constipation, leaky gut syndrome, and dysbiosis. These herbs include meadowsweet, marshmallow root, licorice root, and flaxseed. The inner gel of aloe species plants is also useful in this regard. Many authorities will also cite slippery elm inner bark; I do not want to downplay the importance of this plant, but currently it is on the endangered list, so we are advised not to use it at the present time.

Diagnostic questions
(these questions assess the level of risk of the mixed biliary type)

▷ Do you easily feel full and bloated, even when you haven't really eaten much?

▷ Do you experience any nausea associated with eating rich, fatty foods?

▷ Do you experience any cravings for sweet foods?

▷ Are you ever constipated?

▷ Do you notice that your digestion suffers under stress?

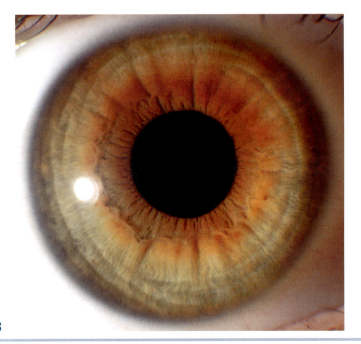

FIGURE 3.13

Mixed iris.

Positive suggestions for the mixed type

▷ Your digestion is your greatest ally: its symptoms are messages intended to guide you to correct eating patterns.

▷ Listening to your digestion can also guide your life choices, through the phenomenon of "gut instinct".
(See Figure 3.13.)

NOTES

1. Larsson, M., Pedersen, N., & Stattin, H. (2007). Associations between iris characteristics and personality in adulthood. *Biological Psychology, 75*: 165–175.
2. Markle, A. (1976). Eye color and responsiveness to arousing stimuli. *Perceptual and Motor Skills, 43*: 127–133.

4

The iridology dispositions: structure types

The first thing you notice about someone's irides is their color. You do not generally notice their texture, because the features are usually extremely small. However, with good light, the irides' features can be seen even with the naked eye; with a small amount of magnification, they reveal the elements by which you can read a person's true individuality. (See Figure 4.1.)

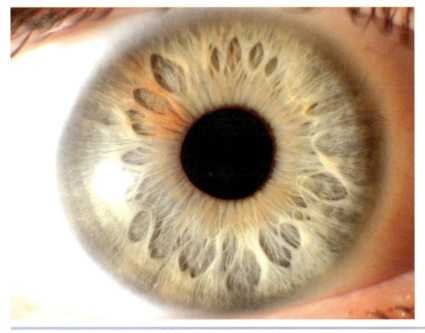

FIGURE 4.1

An example of an individual "open" iris structure.

In this chapter, I outline a classification system that differentiates between commonly seen structural types and their meanings in terms of physiological function and the energetic behavior of the body. The classification originated with Josef Deck and was further developed by Willy Hauser, Josef Karl, and Rudolph Stolz.

This approach can be useful, but there are limitations. First, it does not include people who display composite features—a mixture of more than one type—and, second, it relies too much on a valuation of strength without noting compensatory factors. It assumes that a strong constitution is desirable and a weak constitution automatically portends trouble. This is, as we shall see, far from the truth.

The term given to this aspect of a person's constitution is *disposition*. It may be considered the second level of iris constitutional analysis, after the color types. We will see that, in addition to highlighting certain physiological concerns, this category also reveals character tendencies and typical behavioral responses to the world and to life.

It may not always be possible to assign a structural type to a person. Many people have a mixture of tighter and looser areas of structure within their irides. In these cases, you should look at the individual indications as they are displayed and, with the help of an iris chart (see chapter 6), make assessments concerning specific organs and pathways in the body, according to what you see. (Some guidance on this is given in Chapter 7.)

We look at five basic types, while noting that they do not cover variation. In describing these types, I have departed from the accepted iridology language, for two reasons: one, the language itself can be unhelpfully negative, and I do not wish to place negative connotations in the minds of my patients. Two, the titles I have chosen represent certain functional and behavioral adaptations that can actually be seen in a positive light, even though each may have its risk factors. I have, however, included the original iridology language for your education and information, while commenting on the subject in a more balanced way.

To assist with understanding of the structural types, remember that the iris consists of connective tissue and is thereby considered to represent or mirror connective-tissue integrity throughout the organism. A key word here is *resistance*: structural integrity of the iris is a measure of the resistance of the organism, and of individual parts, or organs, within the organism. Resistance is usually thought of as akin to immunity, which indeed it is; however, let us not make the mistake of assuming that "high" resistance is always to be desired. We will see that it cuts both ways: the high- and the low-resistance types each have their strengths and their weaknesses. Each type represents a specific adaptation in the face of the stresses and threats endemic to life on earth.

The five basic structural types:

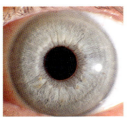

1. *High-resistance type:* finely arranged, high-density fiber structure

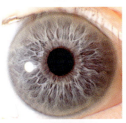

2. *Flexible–adaptive type:* loosely arranged, low-density fiber structure

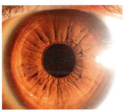

3. *Self-protective type:* presence of deep furrows within the iris

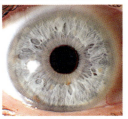

4. *Hormone-regulatory type:* low-density tissue in the hormonal zone

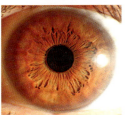

5. *Digestion-regulatory type:* low-density tissue in the digestive zone

Fiber structure

When discussing the structural element of constitution, the older style of iridology often refers—mistakenly, I believe—only to the density of the iris, describing a fine, closely arranged fiber structure as a "silk" constitution, implying greater constitutional strength. The lower the grade of iris texture, the "weaker" the constitution, and the greater the disposition to pathology or disease. The grades may be described as silk, linen, net, and hessian (Figure 4.2). The disadvantage of this is that if you are a "lower grade" type, it is automatically implied that you are at greater risk of pathology. This, as I have indicated above, is not true, and we will see why as we go along.

THE HIGH-RESISTANCE IRIS

Known also within iridology as the neurogenic type, this iris indicates a so-called strong constitution, and it is associated with higher-than-average levels of energy, stamina, and endurance. The keynote of people with irides of this type is resistance. (See Figure 4.3.)

Neurogenic: a definition

"Forming, originating in, or controlled by nervous tissue; induced or modified by nervous factors; disordered because of abnormally altered neural relations." [Merriam-Webster Dictionary]

This iris type is characterized by a dense, closely arranged fiber structure. The fibers throughout the stroma are fine and packed together, containing few if any openings or "lacunae." This iris structure was once thought to be specific to the blue-eyed type; we can, however, readily observe it in all three color types. Although it is important to be able to see the fibers clearly in order to accurately assess the texture, in the darkly pigmented types we can assume the high-resistance type where the

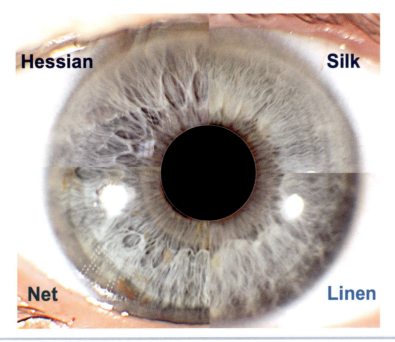

Hessian

Silk

Net

Linen

FIGURE 4.2

Composite showing different grades of iris texture.

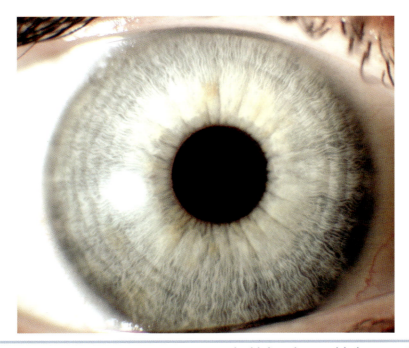

FIGURE 4.3

The high-resistance iris (neurogenic disposition).

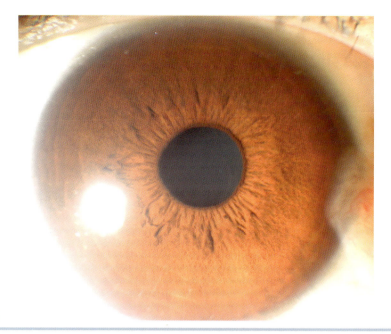

FIGURE 4.4

Dark brown high-resistance iris (hematogenic neurogenic).

surface of the iris is completely smooth, with very few features. (Figure 4.4.)

Density of the iris is regarded as a measure of the ability to resist threats presented by pathogens (bacteria, viruses, etc.) and other invading material. Therefore, people of this type often excel in immune capacity and strength. Rheumatic-type people (see "The Lymphatic Constitution," in Chapter 3) frequently fall into this structural category.

However, there is a need for caution. Because of higher levels of energy and stamina, there is frequently a tendency to overdo things and drive oneself too hard, and consequently these individuals are more susceptible to "crash and burn." I have seen more chronic fatigue syndrome in so-called strong iris types than in so-called weaker ones.

Characteristic tendencies

"Strong" iris types are frequently found among care workers and those in caring roles—for example, the tireless mother who holds the family together and on whom everyone relies. Equally, it describes the businessman or businesswoman working late into the evening, seldom taking time out with their families or taking holidays and relying too much on caffeine to stimulate the adrenal glands.

Strong iris types tend to leave little time to relax and so have less opportunity to discharge accumulated stress. The presence of even *one* lacuna ("weakness" marking), for example, may be said to represent the safety valve in a pressure cooker: without it, there is going to be an explosion—or, possibly, an implosion. Because of this, they may eventually hit the brick wall harder than most when the time comes. Most people with this pattern need to learn to slow down, relax, take breaks, and find ways of dispersing the pressure.

Energetically, these people are kinesthetic types: they are action-oriented and practical. They can also be very sensitive and may tend to hold a lot inside and not process their emotions fully, so that these build up, adding to the pressure. However, generally they do not have time for lengthy deliberations, or for indulging sensitive feelings, focused as they are upon results and problem-solving.

Their sensitivity is, however, responsible for their powerful focus on outcomes and goals. Acutely aware of, and intimately affected by, the great well of suffering in the world, they are externally and altruistically oriented, passionately driven to make the world a better place for all. While there is still suffering and pain, they must fix it, however misguided this may sometimes appear to others.

Their strong capacity for resistance has both positive and negative effects. As well as resisting damaging pathological factors, they can also resist positive influences. It may be difficult to give them advice, because they think they know best, and they sometimes cannot listen. Gaining the attention of and motivating a high-resistance individual is best achieved through the use of practical demonstrations, or by instructing them in hands-on experience. Otherwise in the consulting room their minds will be highly likely to be running ahead, planning the rest of their day, and their attention will readily wander onto the myriad problems or projects that they are dealing with at any one time. I have been known to take such people into the kitchen and get them physically involved in making a herbal tea, or a liver flush: that is something they won't forget!

If the nerves and adrenals can be maintained and supported adequately, people of this type can be the most efficient and productive in any workforce. However, they are susceptible to overextending and may, as a result, suffer from disorders of the nervous system, from minor cramps and ticks, through neuroses and depression, to more serious neuropathies, such as multiple sclerosis or Parkinsonism. One of their most dangerous traits is their apparent ability to ignore and override symptoms when they do occur, thus increasing the risk of pathology overtaking them unawares.

Within this category, there are two subtypes: the high-resistance sensitive type, and the high-resistance robust type.

High-resistance–sensitive type (sensitive neurogenic)

This type accounts for the majority of high-resistance types. These people are strong, but they have a tendency toward worry and anxiety. They have finely tuned nervous systems and are vulnerable to harsh or intrusive stimuli—including the negative emotions of people around them, which they are finely tuned to intercept.

High-resistance–sensitive types have very fine iris fibers, closely packed, and with a very fine "silk" texture. But their collarette is much less prominent than that of the high-resistance–robust type and sometimes almost invisible. There may be circular features, "contraction furrows": ripple-like grooves around the iris disk. (See Figure 4.5.)

High-resistance–robust type (robust neurogenic)

The term "adrenalin junkie" can describe this type. These people tend toward feats of physical endurance and daring, with little regard for personal safety. They find it hard to relax unless pushed to the limit, and they often choose extreme sports to unwind, using the endorphin release following the output of adrenalin.

People of this type have dense but somewhat coarser-textured (linen rather than silk) irides than their sensitive counterparts. The surface layer of the iris stroma has a wavy appearance, often described as "combed hair," as it stretches out from the collarette to the edge of the iris. The collarette is prominent and often bright white in color, indicating hyperactivity of the autonomic nervous system. (See Figure 4.6.)

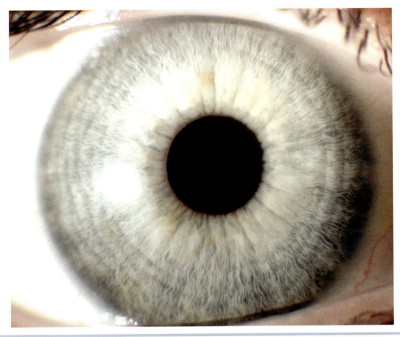

FIGURE 4.5

High-resistance sensitive type (sensitive neurogenic).

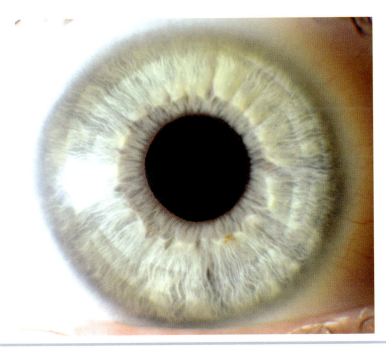

FIGURE 4.6

High-resistance robust type (robust neurogenic).

Living with a high-resistance disposition

Tendencies and risk factors of the type

> "living on one's nerves," sometimes exceeding their resilience;

> workaholic tendencies—difficulty in knowing when to stop and rest, play, eat, etc.;

> overconcern for the welfare of others, constantly "on duty";

> can overtax nerves and adrenal glands resulting in exhaustion;

> prone to actual neuropathies over time.

Dietary needs

Nerve-building foods: Magnesium- and calcium-rich foods—dark-green leafy vegetables, nuts and seeds, fresh fruits; freshly pressed, organic juices.

Omega 3-rich foods: Oily fish, walnuts, flaxseeds.

Whole grains: A highly useful food class for high-resistance people; always choose whole grains, such as oats, barley, buckwheat, and quinoa.

Foods to be avoided

Sugar and caffeine   Since you have a high energy consumption, carbohydrates are in big demand, but do not be tempted to compromise health by overindulging in refined carbohydrates and caffeine: these will lift energy levels for a short period but will not sustain them and will have undesirable long-term consequences. It may be difficult to give these up, and you will need to use strategies such as visualizations or meditation, stretching exercises, or deep breathing (see Chapter 10). Substituting water or a herbal drink for tea and coffee, and fruit and nuts to replace sugar and high-calorie snacks, may help.

Beware of the "caffeine–alcohol" seesaw: can't get going in

the morning without that cup of coffee; can't wind down in the evening without half a bottle of wine! Choose some nice, nerve-nourishing herbal teas instead of the latter, and try a warming grain coffee substitute for the former.

A healthy lifestyle

Relax: Pace yourself, to ensure that you make the most of your above-average strength and endurance. You are rarely still, either physically or mentally, so use exercise routines such as yoga or Tai Chi to help you to relax.

Ensure sufficiency and quality of sleep: Sleep is the mother of all regenerative tonics, and you may tend to shortchange yourself on this precious commodity. If you are typically restless or troubled at night, address this as a priority.

Learn to say "No":   You need to refuse to do things occasionally, to prevent yourself becoming overcommitted. Even though you can accomplish most tasks faster than other people, you must learn to restrain yourself.

Look after yourself: Most high-resistance-type people (especially high-resistance–robust types) are irritated by illness and don't have time for it. You may tend to resort to painkillers to smother symptoms and ignore them. You can do this for years and not notice the wear and tear, but you may pay for it later with more serious symptoms.

Learn to love yourself: You are your own harshest critic and are much better at looking after others than yourself. You are deserving of unconditional love, just as you are!

Be prepared to make lifestyle changes: If healing is to be achieved, you must commit to lifestyle changes. If you cause a relapse of an illness, it may be more difficult to recover in subsequent times. Illness often needs to be addressed by reevaluating your lifestyle.

Supportive exercise

Because of your reserves of strength and stamina, you tend to like vigorous exercise, and you may feel the need to exert yourself. Exercise is also a very efficient way of maintaining health and balance within the nerve system. Aerobic exercise is powered by the sympathetic nervous system, and there is an automatic synergistic reaction, whereby, after exercising, the parasympathetic nervous system assumes dominance through the release of the hormone endorphin, which is chemically similar to opiates. This "endorphin kick" calms, relaxes, and stills the body and mind. Activities such as meditation are easier for you after vigorous exercise.

Herbal choices

Nerve builders and nourisher: In herbal medicine, we call these "nervous trophorestoratives," which means that they nourish and strengthen the nervous system. Use wild oats, vervain, skullcap, and ashwagandha. Valerian is also an excellent source of calcium— a mineral used in large quantities by the nervous system—but beware, valerian is a "hot" herb that can overstimulate already overheated people!

Relaxants and antispasmodics: These are particularly useful at the end of the day for taking the tone of things down a notch or two. Make a relaxing evening tea with lime blossom, passionflower, skullcap, or chamomile, and add a touch of lavender flowers and rose petals for color, aromatic fragrance, and additional feel-good factor.

Stress busters and stamina builders: The so-called adaptogens are also adrenal tonics and work to restore the whole system when under pressure or chronic stress. Although you may feel you thrive on stress (many neurogenics do), you can easily overdo it. Use ginseng (any variety), wild oats, astragalus, licorice, ashwagandha.

Diagnostic questions
(these questions assess the level of risk of the high-resistance type)

> Do you find it difficult to shut down and turn off after work?
> Are you always three steps ahead of yourself, or compulsively multitasking?
> Is your sleep short, restless, or disturbed?
> Do you frequently find yourself "running on empty"?
> Are you always the last person you look after or take care of?

Positive suggestions for the high-resistance type

> Your strength and endurance is legendary: others are lucky to have you in their lives, watching their backs.
> Looking after Number One is not selfish: it is necessary. How are you going to do everything you need to do if you are exhausted and sick? (See Figure 4.7.)

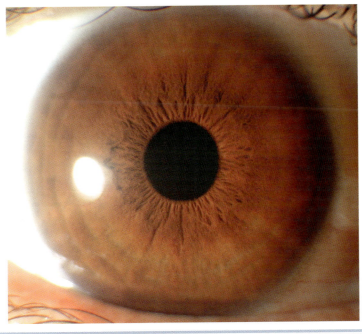

FIGURE 4.7

Dark mixed high-resistance type (mixed biliary neurogenic).

THE FLEXIBLE–ADAPTIVE IRIS

At the opposite extreme from the high-density, high-resistance type are people of the low-density, flexible–adaptive type, known in iridology terminology as the connective-tissue weakness type. (See Figure 4.8.)

The flexible–adaptive disposition is shown by a low-density iris, where the fibers are far less numerous than those in the high-resistance-iris type. The color is therefore darker, as the dark color of the base leaf is more visible through rarefied fibers, with the exception of sometimes very bright *individual* fibers, which often provide a compensatory strength or reactivity. The stroma of the iris is therefore more penetrable than in other types. This means that more light can enter the inner levels of the iris and stimulate reflex sites and nerve endings, which may be an advantageous evolutionary adaptation strategy in the case of actual connective-tissue compromise.

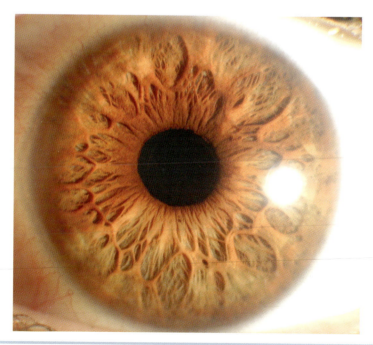

FIGURE 4.8

The flexible-adaptive iris (connective tissue weakness disposition).

While this iris type was also originally considered specific to people with blue eyes, the quality of greater openness can apply to all iris color types, as Figure 4.8 demonstrates.

Traditionally, areas of open structure have been regarded as indicative of weakness in the organs linked reflexively to the site and should be taken seriously as targets for treatment. Because it is pervasive throughout the irides, this openness implies a less robust constitution than others, particularly that of the high-resistance-iris type, and yet its receptivity may also be considered its chief advantage.

The high-resistance type's close-textured iris is responsible for its emphasis on resistance, but this can come at the cost of some stubbornness and resistance to change. The reverse is true of the flexible–adaptive persons. They do not resist well and are nominally at higher risk of attracting damaging pathological influences; however, they also know themselves well enough to make whatever adaptations in lifestyle are necessary to preserve health to its optimum capacity.

Reflecting the open structure of their irides, people of this type are also emotionally and mentally open and receptive in a positive way and are likely, on that account, to be among those who are most attentive to others. This is one reason why I discourage the use of the standard term *connective-tissue weakness*: it sends a message of inferiority to people who are likely to be extremely sensitive to this. Emphasizing flexibility and adaptability is positive and validating, and that is equally going to be received and taken to heart.

Characteristic tendencies

Flexible–adaptive people rely on energy conservation and prudence. Conscious of their limits, they will pull back from overstretching and retire to regenerate. Knowing that they do not heal as easily as others, they will not readily put themselves in dangerous situations. However, when pressured, these people's openness is an advantage. In difficult situations, keeping one's ears and eyes open is a good strategy for survival. In fact, Farida Sharan, an iridologist and natural healer, dubbed this the "survivor–adjuster" type.[1]

Physiologically, they may tend to suffer from connective-tissue disorders, including being prone to injury—for example, in a sporting situation—and hypermobility of joints. Deficiency of connective tissue may also result in the prolapse of organs—for example, of the uterus, bowel, or bladder.

There may be difficulty in transporting oxygen and nutrients to where they are needed, and drainage may be poor, resulting in retention of fluids (edema) and tissue encumbrance with retained toxins.

Flexible–adaptive people need to look after themselves, and they are usually aware of this. Receptivity is key for these "open" people. They readily respond to advice, and their accentuated auditory sensitivity means that audiotapes, music, and chanting all can be used with greater benefit and efficacy in healing than for some other types. As noted above, this extends to the very words one uses when dealing with them—and how one speaks to them. (See Figure 4.9.)

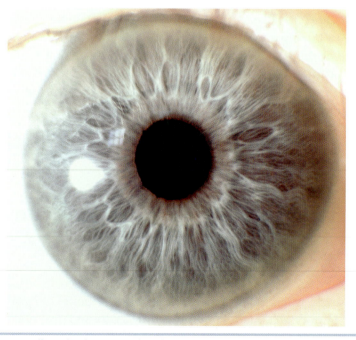

FIGURE 4.9

Flexible-adaptive type (lymphatic connective tissue weakness).

Living with a flexible–adaptive disposition

The true connective-tissue receptive iris is relatively rare, and there are degrees of openness within people of this type. It is perfectly possible for them to live in harmony with their constitution.

Tendencies and risk factors of the type

> ▷ less robust constitutions, greater susceptibility to invasive influences;
>
> ▷ less robust connective tissue, prone to weak ligaments, easy injury, etc.;
>
> ▷ greater need for immune support: antioxidants and micronutrients;
>
> ▷ greater need for self-care, but self-awareness and flexibility of approach generally compensates.

Dietary needs

Fresh produce: Eat plenty of fruit and vegetables rich in essential nutrients such as vitamins, especially those high in vitamin C, minerals, trace elements, and antioxidants. Oranges, blackcurrants, strawberries, potatoes, brussels sprouts, broccoli, green leafy vegetables, green peppers, and parsley are all good choices.

Detoxification: Eat foods that gently assist elimination and do not add to toxic residues, such as fresh fruit (high in vitamin C, antioxidants, and water content). In addition to the fruit and vegetables listed above, all red fruits (such as blackberries, raspberries, redcurrants, bilberries, and cranberries), and fruit and vegetable juices, are ideal. Juicing maximizes the mineral and vitamin absorption from the foods juiced. Also, certain "superfoods," such as spirulina, chlorella, and alfalfa, are beneficial.

A healthy lifestyle

Time to relax and regenerate: Connective-tissue receptive individuals tend to have less stamina than others and should not be pushed too hard. If this is your type, make sure you allow sufficient time for relaxation and recuperation after any strenuous activity or period. Take care that your lifestyle does not demand too much of you. Learn to measure your pace and find creative ways to adapt to the demands of life.

Supportive exercise

Core strengthening is key to the health of this type—hatha yoga, pilates, and free weights encourage the development of postural integrity and compensatory muscular strength. Swimming is the best form of aerobic exercise. Practice walking at a relaxed pace, preferably on grass or bare earth, sand, and so forth (to avoid skeletal shock).

Avoid sports or activities that involve high musculoskeletal impact: I once read the irides of a 12-year-old boy who had got into King's College London on a rugby scholarship. I warned his mother to take great care of his nutrition and to attend promptly to the healing of injuries. Nonetheless, a year later she mournfully related that I had been correct: he had had to change to cricket!

Herbal choices

Immunity stimulants and protectors: Echinacea, elder, elecampane, eucalyptus, garlic, schisandra, wild indigo, and wild cherry.

Stamina-building: Take adaptogens: astragalus, Siberian ginseng, oat seed, ashwagandha.

Healing and strengthening connective tissue: Vulnerary herbs, such as comfrey (generally not advised for internal use but can be used topically on injuries), horsetail (high in organic silica, which can be converted by the body to calcium), and gotu kola (a general healer and strengthener known to improve collagen synthesis).

Detoxifying: Detoxify slowly, using diet as the foundation. Use local herbs, such as dandelion, nettle, cleavers, red clover, dock, and burdock.

Diagnostic questions
(these questions assess the level of risk of a flexible–adaptive type)

▷ Do you need to take frequent breaks for regrouping and healing?

▷ Are you susceptible to frequent musculoskeletal injury?

▷ Do you easily become lethargic and out of sorts if you do not live healthily?

▷ Are you unusually susceptible to negative or unkind comments from others?

Positive suggestions for the flexible–adaptive type

▷ What you may lack in stamina and strength, you more than make up for in flexibility and resourcefulness.

▷ You always know best how to heal yourself.
(See Figure 4.10.)

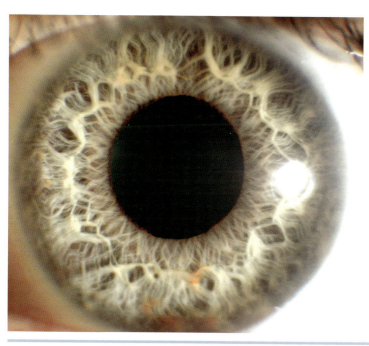

FIGURE 4.10

A further example of a flexible adaptive type.

THE SELF-PROTECTIVE IRIS

Self-protective people are related to high-resistance individuals, both having dense irides. The type is identified by a tell-tale pattern of deep circular and radial furrows within the iris disk. They construct highly effective defenses, often physical, which allow them to focus and screen out unwanted information. (See Figure 4.11.)

The correct iridological name for this type is *larvate tetanic.* "Larvate" comes from a Latin word that originally translates as "mask" (and is the same root as that which gives rise to "larva," in the sense of a pupating insect); "tetanic" means "spasm" or "contraction" (same origin for the medical term *tetany,* and the pathology known as *tetanus*). In other words, this type forms a protective mask by means of maintaining patterns of physical tension, sometimes also known as "body armor."

Like individuals of the high-resistance type, these people are kinesthetic and solution-oriented. They are frequently seen as exhibiting calm, rational behavior that inspires confidence. The characteristic iris features of self-protective people include contraction (circular) furrows—at least three- or four-deep concentric circular grooves in the iris—and radial furrows. The latter can be major radials: deep troughs that radiate outward from the pupil margin, cutting through the border of the collarette, into the outer part of the iris disk; or they can be minor radials: smaller and less deep, which start at the border of the collarette. (See Figure 4.12.)

Characteristic tendencies

Self-protective people, like high-resistance individuals, may be driven by anxiety. The defenses also represent fear and anxiety, leading to a need for withdrawal and self-protection/self-preservation. A confident exterior frequently masks a vulnerable inner world, and the protective patterns shield them from an environment that is perceived (usually unconsciously) as harsh and threatening. Another name for these types is the *"anxiety tetanic."*

A client of mine, an award-winning poet, had this iris pattern. I said to her once, "It's like you're in a state of permanent

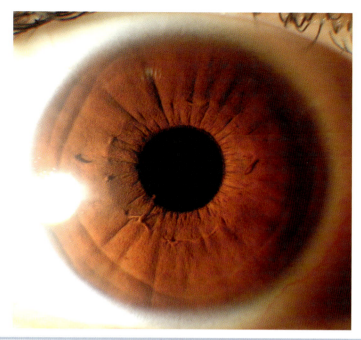

FIGURE 4.11

The self-protective iris (larvate tetanic disposition).

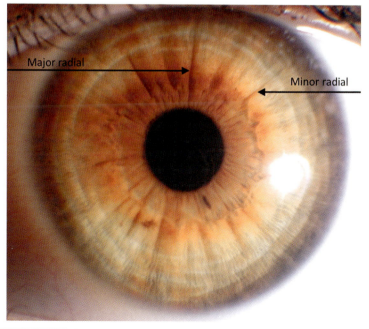

FIGURE 4.12

Mixed biliary self-protective iris illustrating radial furrow types.

emergency." She resonated strongly with the expression, and it became the title of her next volume of poems.

The idea behind this is that the adrenal system—in fact, the entire hypothalamus–pituitary–adrenal complex (the HPA axis)—is in a continual state of hypervigilance: in other words, the sympathetic nerve response is chronically dominant, and there is a certain tendency to secrete higher than normal amounts of the stress hormone, cortisol. This can be observed at the start of the day—when cortisol is highest, and when they are often up with the lark and ready to go, way ahead of most other people.

However, self-protective people are also generally extremely socially aware and gregarious: the radial furrows, like sun rays, represent openness and generosity. The circular furrows denote an "autonomic" habit of strategic withdrawal and self-concealment, helping them to perform with confidence, keeping people unaware of their sensitivity. On the one hand, there is openness; on the other, there is retreat. To say that they often have a *superficial* physical beauty and attractiveness would be to suggest that they are somehow deceiving us: in fact, they are extremely genuine people, but they have perfected the trick of keeping their vulnerable core safe and hidden behind a highly effective, and attractive, social exterior.

I have occasionally likened them to the swan that glides across the pond, seemingly serene and elegant, yet no one sees the hard work being done paddling beneath the surface. People of this type can suffer in silence, their pain and their struggle generally unacknowledged, because unseen, by others.

Self-protective people always go back to their own space at the end of the day for regrouping, and are usually insistent upon regular patterns of sleeping and eating in order to ensure adequate energy and resources for the following day's exertions. In a way, the regular radial furrows around the entire disk of the iris are reminiscent of a clock face, keeping strict time to regulate their activities. They may easily become disorientated if their routines are upset or delayed.

Physiologically, self-protective individuals also resemble high-resistance people. However, the maintenance of patterns of muscular contractions—a part of their defensive reactions—demands large amounts of energy. There is increased pressure on gastrointestinal dynamics to supply this energy. This, combined with the presence of radial furrows, which cut through the collarette and indicate that the nerve supply to the digestive organs may be affected, points to the potential for a damaging "energy gap" to appear, especially under stress. Additionally, they will tend to feel their stress in their stomach and intestines, often experiencing a knot of tension in that location—yet another name for the type is *anxiety gastric*. People of this type frequently suffer from tension and pain, but they respond well to massage and physical therapies. Cramps (including, for women, menstrual cramps), tics, spasms, and neuromuscular tension are also common.

Because of the high demand for energy and the potential for digestive compromise, self-protective individuals can develop a widening "energy gap" as the years go by, which can sometimes lead to premature feelings of exhaustion, fatigue, and enervation. The good news is that once the dynamics causing this are understood and intercepted, it is relatively easily corrected: upregulate digestion, downregulate the HPA "stress" response.

This iris type is most frequently found among the hematogenic and mixed iris colors, which emphasize the need to care for gastrointestinal health. The pattern is, however, increasingly found also in lymphatic irides.

Living with a self-protective disposition

Tendencies and risk factors of the type

➤ outer protective layer maintained by neuromuscular tension—"body armor"—which depletes energy by means of high demand for certain nutrients;

➤ high demand for energy but low energy provision, as tension also adversely affects digestion;

➤ may hide inner vulnerability behind a "mask," frequently seen as calm and in control, even when anxious;

➤ need for regularity and recuperative space in daily routine—working, eating, sleeping.

Dietary needs

Juices, smoothies, and "superfoods":   These supply a high amount of essential nutrients, especially those required for a healthy nervous system.

Nerve builders: Like the high-resistance type, you need to eat foods that nourish your nervous system. Such foods will be high in B vitamins and will include whole grains, nutritional yeast, wheat germ, beansprouts, avocados, nuts, mushrooms, and green leafy vegetables. You also need to take more calcium, which is found in green vegetables, oranges, almonds, and tofu, and the cofactors essential for the absorption of calcium, such as vitamins A and C, found in citrus fruit and berries, and magnesium (Nature's "chill-out" mineral), found in nuts, bananas, and soya beans.

Kidney strengtheners: The kidneys are regarded as the seat of vitality in traditional medicine, and they can be regarded as the foundation of good energy and resistance. In Western medical speak they correspond to the adrenals, and there is a very close interaction between the adrenals and the nerves. Support the kidneys with pulses, barley grain, barley grass (add to smoothies), and add warmth through cooked food.

A healthy lifestyle

Balance: Measured rest and work ratios are essential. There is an inherent desire for order and routine, which can, under duress, sometimes present as excessive or even obsessive. Overdrawing on your reserves can have serious consequences. Ensure sufficiency of sleep, regular meals in a relaxed space, and time for recreation and socializing.

Care of digestion: The suggestions offered in the section on the mixed iris type should be studied carefully by those of this type, as they will be beneficial.

Massage: Treat yourself to a massage or bodywork session as frequently as you can. Your tendency to muscular tension will need to be eased and soothed on a regular basis.

Epsom salts (magnesium sulphate) baths: The relaxing effect of magnesium salts is one of the benefits of bathing in Epsom salts, in addition to its detoxifying effects. Use at least 500g of the salts in the hottest bath you can tolerate. For best results, take a brief cold dip or cold shower to finish—to close down the pores and conserve heat in the interior.

Time for contemplation and reflection: Getting out into Nature is an excellent way to get past constant mental chatter and activity, and fear and apprehension. It helps bypass the rational mind and helps achieve deep levels of relaxation.

Supportive exercise

You may find goal-oriented exercise, such as weight training and competitive activities, attractive, but you should guard against exercise becoming too regimented and obsessional. There is also a need to let go into more creative modes, so dance is an excellent form of exercise for you. Middle Eastern or Arabic dance styles (*Raqs Sharqi*—"Dance of the East"), and Gabrielle Roth's "5Rhythms" dance cycle are ideal.

Herbal choices

Nervines and antispasmodics: Especially good are wild oat, skullcap, and vervain. Lime blossom, cramp bark, and black cohosh also relieve muscular tension. (See also the suggestions for the high-resistance type.)

Digestion-supporting: Bitter tonics and carminatives support your digestion and ensure you get a maximum uptake of nutrients. (See the suggestions for the mixed type.)

Adaptogens: Siberian ginseng, astragalus, wild oat, ashwagandha, and schisandra improve stamina and tone the adrenals.

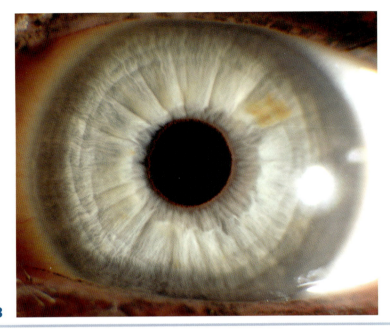

FIGURE 4.13

Self-protective iris (lymphatic larvate tetanic).

Diagnostic questions

(these questions assess the level of risk of a self-protective type)

▷ Are you aware of high levels of tension affecting your muscles?

▷ Is maintaining a strict daily routine important to you—are you, for example, "early to bed, early to rise"?

▷ Do you fear that others will "see through" you to your failings and unworthiness?

▷ Do you carry or experience your stress in your guts?

▷ Do you suffer from debilitating levels of anxiety or irrational fears?

Positive suggestions for the self-protective type:

▷ People love you, no matter what you believe your failings to be.

▷ You have excellent people skills, which will generally get you exactly where you want to be—if you let them!

(See Figure 4.13.)

THE HORMONE-REGULATORY IRIS

The glands central to this iris type are the endocrine organs, whose function is to regulate metabolic activity through the release of hormones. The type is identified by a flower-petal-like appearance of lacunae encircling the border of the collarette. It is found in all color types. (Figure 4.14.)

Another term describing people of this type is their polyglandular disposition: the glands referred to are the endocrine, or hormonal, glands. The prefix "poly-" (meaning many) carries the suggestion that if one gland is functioning abnormally, others may also be affected. The glandular system works as a unit; the pituitary or master gland, in the brain, directs the rest of the organs or glands elsewhere in the body. This is often referred to as the "endocrine orchestra," with the pituitary gland considered as the conductor. Many hormonal activities are triggered by signals from the pituitary. The emphasis here on harmony and balance is significant for this disposition, who frequently struggle to find a stable norm between high amplitudes of mood and energy.

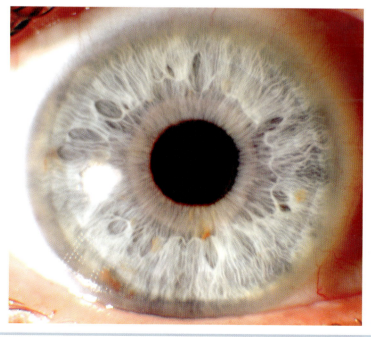

FIGURE 4.14

The hormone-regulatory iris (polyglandular disposition).

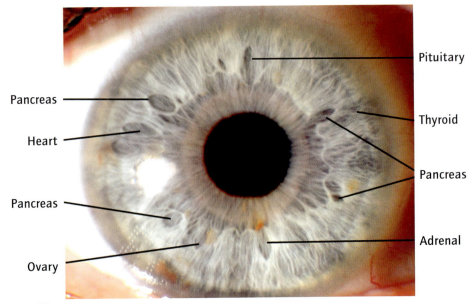

Pituitary

Pancreas

Thyroid

Heart

Pancreas

Pancreas

Adrenal

Ovary

FIGURE 4.15

The hormone-regulatory iris showing positions of the major endocrine organs.

The area immediately outside the border of the collarette is known as the *humoral zone* (see Chapter 6) and refers to the deep body fluids—blood, and lymph—but it is also known as the *hormonal zone*, as this is the zone in which the major hormonal organs—the pituitary, the adrenals, the gonads, and the pancreas—are found in the iris chart. Interrupted iris texture in this area suggests a potential for a disruption in, or instability of, hormone function. (Figure 4.15.)

Characteristic tendencies

Individuals with a hormone-regulatory disposition are capable of tremendous creative energetic output, but will occasionally experience slumps of energy and motivation. These will be short-lived and reflect a temporary need to recalibrate and rejuvenate. They are strongly emotionally driven and tend to wear their hearts on their sleeves—what you see is exactly what you get (in contrast, perhaps, to the self-protective type). They can flow effortlessly between a wide range of emotional responses, but mood swings can be a problem. Open spaces in the iris also denote receptivity, as also for the flexible–adaptive type, and these people resonate readily with others, are great listeners, and can be highly creative.

Physiologically, people of this type may suffer from hormonal complaints. The tendency toward erratic functioning of the endocrine glands can portend problems with energy management, as well as difficulty stabilizing emotions and mood. Women of this type may be more vulnerable to menopausal difficulties, especially if the glands have been overworked during life up to that point. The health of the adrenal glands, especially, is vital to a smooth transit through the female change of life.

Among other pathologies frequently experienced are thyroid difficulties, adrenal instability and exhaustion, and Type 2 diabetes, the latter being especially common in people of the mixed and hematogenic-iris types. A tendency early in life to hypoglycemia can warn of a later potential for diabetes if it is not addressed; an overactive thyroid can become underactive later; a tendency to hyperactivity of the adrenals may become chronic fatigue. Thus, unmanaged activity early in life can lead to exhaustion later. Work is needed to restore balance and moderation, and this will prolong the life of the organs concerned. In particular, work to stabilize blood sugar crashes, which are not uncommon, especially after lunch or in the early afternoon.

Digestion is crucial in maintaining good operation of the hormonal glands, and taking bitter tonics to stimulate digestion will help achieve this. Part of the understanding that informs this is that the humoral zone in which these signs are found is also the zone of transportation and distribution of nutrients: it is positioned immediately outside the digestive ring and may be regarded as the first stage reached by nutriment converted in the digestive crucible in its metabolic journey to nourish, energize, and regenerate the entire organism. From this central ring, nutrients are transported across various membranes into the deep-level blood circulation and onward to the whole system. There is an old trick, in Western herbal medicine, of using the bitter tonics (see above), specifically to stimulate and regulate the hormonal system.

Being predominantly emotionally driven, hormone-regulatory types will frequently appear changeable or even unreliable to others: the person you get today may not be the person you get tomorrow! To themselves, however, this is just normal: why would you try to be the same person, with the same opinions, preferences, and priorities, all the time, when you have such a wealth of possibilities available to you in terms of emotional response? In many ways, this guards against any tendency toward stagnation and "stuckness," and these types, like the flexible–adaptive types with whom they have this in common, tend to be open-minded and flexible in their approach to life.

In fact, they thrive on variety and the endless ebb and flow of feelings and impressions. They will easily get bored if forced to sit at a desk all day, and the advice for them, should they have made this somewhat incongruous choice in life, is that they should at least get up and move, change focus, even change activities, if possible, on a regular basis. They function better in what used to be called the intuitive and inspirational "right brain" than in the logical and analytical "left brain," and hence the link with creativity. If they can be disciplined enough (a big "if" in some cases!), then their creativity and imagination can be globally encompassing and universally inspiring.

Out of balance, however, there are some significant dangers, particularly of addiction. The quest for new sensations, the boredom and ennui of "ordinary life," can propel hormone-regulatory types into negative and self-indulgent habits, from which it may be difficult to extract themselves. The answer, as always, is to be found in seeking moderation and balance—not in terms of homogeneity, but in the judicious selection of activities and experiences: addiction can, after all, be the most boring and repetitive state out there! (See Figure 4.16.)

Living with a hormone-regulatory disposition

Tendencies and risk factors of the type

- ▷ erratic hormone levels, leading to erratic energy levels and emotional changeability;
- ▷ tendency toward blood sugar irregularities and hypoglycemia/diabetes;
- ▷ although creative and imaginative, can have difficulties finding stability or consistency;
- ▷ a need for frequent changes of focus in order to maintain interest and energy.

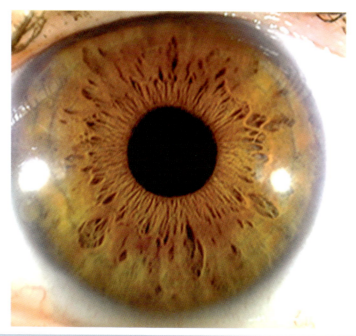

FIGURE 4.16

Mixed hormone regulatory type (mixed biliary polyglandular).

Dietary needs

Mealtime hygiene: The same advice as for the mixed biliary constitution. Optimizing digestion and absorption is key to maintaining the stability and stamina of the endocrine organs.

Bitter tonics and appetizers: Again, similarly to the mixed biliary type, the "priming" of digestion before eating can greatly enhance both the experience and the benefits of nutrition.

A "kidney-friendly" diet: In traditional Chinese medicine (TCM) it is the kidneys, not the brain/pituitary, that are considered to be the governor of endocrine activity—and, by the same token, of fertility and reproduction. In the Western understanding, this equates to the adrenals—which are, after all, tightly involved with the pituitary by means of the HPA axis. The Chinese also regard the kidneys as the seat of our vitality, and the house where our very essence (Jing) is stored.

The color that corresponds to kidney in the Chinese 5-elements system is black: black foods, such as blackberries, black sesame seeds, black beans, seaweeds, black chia seeds, and wild rice can be tried. Pulses generally are considered strengthening to the kidneys—there's a "doctrine of signatures" to be seen there: many pulses are actually shaped like a kidney. Similarly to the diet recommended for weak digestion, warming foods and mild spices may also be used.

Foods to be avoided

Sugars: Reduce consumption of refined and simple sugars like sweets, chocolate (unless raw), biscuits, and cakes. These give energy, but it dissipates quickly. Sugar also puts pressure on the pancreas—a key member of the endocrine system.

Alcohol, caffeine, and stimulants: Because of the hormone-regulatory type's ease of developing addictive patterns, such substances are best avoided. Stimulants can also overtax the adrenals and the thyroid, causing them to get prematurely run down.

A healthy lifestyle

Frequent breaks and avoidance of stagnation: Variable iris texture implies changeable energy patterns. You need frequent breaks at work and plenty of variety of focus. Get up, move around, go outside, read a little, or listen to some music—if possible without getting fired!

Avoid burning the candle at both ends, especially as you get older, however much you may feel like "going with the flow": late nights and partying must be balanced with wholesome food, exercise, and sleep.

Supportive exercise

Yoga, Qi Gong, and Tai Chi all boost the endocrine system. A moderate amount of aerobic exercise is also recommended. Reiki (energy that is channeled through the hands) also can reenergize the endocrine system and help to recharge your batteries.

Herbal choices

Digestion-supporting herbs: Bitter tonics, including gentian, the wormwood family, citrus peel, and Swedish bitters stimulate digestion and absorption.

Endocrine-supporting herbs:

> *Pituitary support:* Dong quai, chaste tree berry, mugwort, ginkgo, St John's wort;
> *Underactive thyroid:* Kelp, nettle, damiana, oat seed, ashwagandha, rosemary;
> *Overactive thyroid:* Bugleweed, valerian, skullcap, oat straw;
> *Pancreas:* Dandelion, burdock, fenugreek, garlic, juniper berry;
> *Adrenals:* Panax ginseng, Siberian ginseng, astragalus, oat seed, burdock, licorice, borage;
> *Male hormones:* ginseng, damiana, ashwagandha, oat seed, sarsaparilla root;
> *Female hormones:* Dong quai, chaste tree berry, false unicorn root, licorice, black cohosh.

Diagnostic questions
(these questions assess the level of risk of the hormone-regulatory type)

> Do you experience erratic energy levels, either over time, or even on the same day?
> Do you suffer crashes in energy or blood sugar?
> Do you feel constrained and restless in your choice of lifestyle or job?
> Is maintaining a strict daily routine difficult for you?
> Do others feed back to you that you are "overemotional" or unduly changeable?

Positive suggestions for the hormone-regulatory type:

> You are an inherently creative and resourceful person.
> Your ability to experience and enjoy a full range of emotions without getting stuck in any of them is to be envied!
> (See Figure 4.17.)

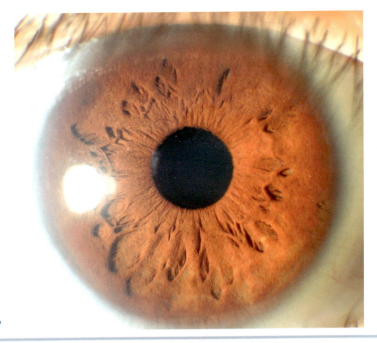

FIGURE 4.17

Dark brown hormone regulatory type (hematogenic polyglandular).

THE DIGESTIVE-REGULATORY IRIS

This type, also known as the gastric disposition, is identified by an expansion of the border of the collarette toward the iris edge, together with loose connective tissue (low-density fiber structure) inside the border (Figure 4.18).

The gastric disposition is in some ways similar to the hormone-regulatory type, of which it may be considered a subtype, and with which it is frequently confused. Common themes include vacillating energy and blood sugar levels, together with suboptimal digestive performance and disturbed gastrointestinal immunity. The focus is on the gastrointestinal tract in all aspects of its function—from the provision of gastric and biliary secretions, through absorption and distribution of nutrients, to immune-related issues such as dysbiosis, parasitic infestation, and leaky gut syndrome, as well as chronic constipation.

Also similarly to the hormone-regulatory type, there is an energetic tendency toward an emotional orientation and an intuitive, rather than analytical, awareness. This is never to say that analysis is not possible, but that it is not the preferred modality in which the world is apprehended or approached. We could use the term "gut instinct," or "gut awareness," implying a cognitive source of information different from that which generally predominates in the current cultural climate.

This may highlight what Michael Gershon referred to as the "second brain"[2]: the existence of the enteric nerve system as a distinct branch of the autonomic nervous system, and the independence of gut awareness from the more familiar—and better validated—intellectual awareness. This type may have an "advance" on data perceived and processed by the gut a long time ahead of it registering with brain-centered consciousness. It may be noted in this context that 70% of the immune system and an estimated 95% of serotonin is located in the gut (leaving just 5% in the brain).

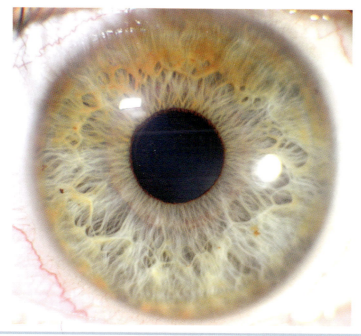

FIGURE 4.18

Digestive-regulatory type (gastric disposition).

Serotonin (5-HT) is associated with mood and is the target for manipulation by so-called "antidepressant" medication, however, its role is actually far more extensive than this suggests, taking in regulatory involvements in immunity, inflammation, metabolic homeostasis, and even bone remodeling—hence the coining of the phrase *digestive-regulatory* to describe this type: so many processes depend on maintaining that all-important gut environment.[3]

Characteristic tendencies

The emphasis for people of this type is clearly on the gastrointestinal tract, and people of this type have predispositions toward indigestion and acid stomach, bloating after eating, constipation, diverticulosis and diverticulitis (the presence of diverticular protrusions in the gut and the possible subsequent inflammation of these), colitis and inflammatory bowel disease (IBD), dysbiosis, and candidosis (disruption of natural gut bacteria and consequent overgrowth of the *Candida albicans* organism).

Parasites are a common problem and may be acquired easily, especially if gut health is not well maintained. The gastric type has a greater need to pay attention to gut immunity to avoid such problems, since the open texture of iris tissue in the digestive reflex area implies less effective defenses against invading organisms. Interestingly, the German iridologist and author, Theodor Kriege,[4] designates areas of multiple lacunae or crypts (*honeycombs*), as "wormnests": this always gets people's attention for the boldness of the assertion, but it makes the point that such areas may, indeed, through disturbed tissue status and immunity, be especially susceptible to parasitic invasion. (See Figure 4.19.)

The type was once referred to as the "abdominal reservoir" type, implying that much is held in the stomach and intestines. This may be literal, as in constipation, but it also may be figurative, as in hanging on to emotions and awareness. Constipation is often associated with a tendency to hang on to the past. On the positive side, this pattern implies greater awareness of the emotional self and relying on "gut instincts."

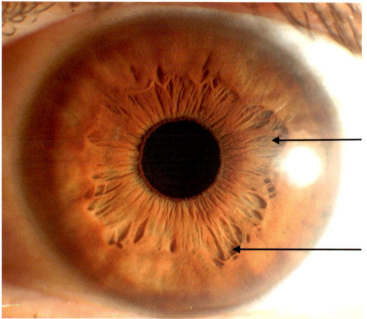

FIGURE 4.19

Mixed gastric type, showing "honeycombs": likely locations for parasitic infestation.

Living with a digestive-regulatory disposition

Tendencies and risk factors of the type

▷ disturbed gastrointestinal immunity, dysbiosis, candidosis, and parasite invasion;

▷ digestive problems of all kinds, ranging from functional insufficiency of secretory organs to chronic inflammatory complains affecting the gastrointestinal mucosa;

▷ tendency toward blood sugar irregularities and hypoglycemia / diabetes;

▷ similar energetic tendencies to the hormone-regulatory type. (See Figure 4.20.)

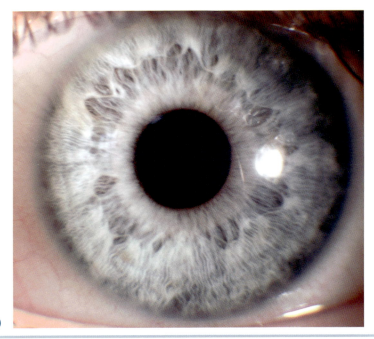

FIGURE 4.20

This person presented with a diagnosis of both Crohn's disease and ulcerative colitis: two major types of inflammatory bowel disease.

Dietary needs

The diet should be clean and unencumbered with processed foods, or with excesses of animal-derived foods—dairy produce, meat, and poultry. These foods will tend to clog the digestive capacity and place unsupportable expectations on it. A plant-based diet is ideal.

Fiber: Eat plenty of whole grains—e.g., organic wholemeal bread or pasta, quinoa, buckwheat—as well as dried peas and beans, fruit, and vegetables. These help to maintain an active bowel motility.

Fruit: Eat plenty of fruit, both fresh and dried, but seek advice on dried fruit if you suspect you have a candida overgrowth. Prunes, figs, and prune juice are good remedies for constipation.

Foods to be avoided

Sugar and refined carbohydrates and fat: These provide only "empty" calories and are not supportive to the digestive system or to health and immunity in general. They may, in addition, end up feeding the pathogens, and not the person. Sugar in particular encourages the growth of negative bacteria and yeasts such as *Candida*.

Animal-derived foods: As mentioned above.

A healthy lifestyle

Much of the advice given for the mixed biliary constitution and the hormone-regulatory type can be usefully employed by the digestive-regulatory individual.

Exercise

The digestive-regulatory type is characteristically predisposed to sluggish digestion and benefits from regular exercise. A walk after mealtimes will greatly help digestion. Do not make this walk too brisk, however, or you may develop cramps.

My favorite exercise for this type is the squat, which works on key energetic principles and may be considered a form of yoga:

The squat

To perform the squat, stand with your feet hip-width apart. You may need to hold onto the back of a chair as you gently lower yourself, bending your knees and keeping your feet flat on the ground if possible. Try bouncing a little to ease yourself down, but do not rise onto the balls of your feet. If you can, go all the way down, flop forward over your knees, clasp your hands at the back of your neck, and gently pull your head down. Breathe deeply into the abdomen—this will stretch you even further. Bounce a little again, easing into the posture and relaxing on the outbreath. Maintain the posture for two to five minutes. Rise slowly and arch your back a little to stretch out in the opposite direction. By compressing and then stretching out the abdomen, you stimulate the internal organs in a gentle fashion.

Herbal choices

Soothing and demulcent: Slippery elm, marshmallow, licorice, linseed, and psyllium husks act as gentle laxatives but also soothe and rebuild the gastrointestinal tract. These are best taken as powders, using one heaped teaspoon mixed with a mug of water or juice, drunk once or twice a day, away from food.

Laxatives and purgatives: Mild laxatives include dandelion root, yellow dock root, and rhubarb root, but for those needing stronger action, herbs such as senna, cascara, and aloe provide sometimes much-needed stimulus to a sluggish or lazy bowel. These herbs work by strongly stimulating the peristaltic motion of the colon, producing regular and easy bowel motions. Caution should be exercised: avoid long-term use, for fear of habituation. These are generally taken in capsules with the last meal of the day, hopefully producing a reliable result first thing the following morning.

Gastrointestinal antiseptics and immune support: Barberry bark, golden seal root, uva ursi leaf, pau d'arco bark, thyme leaf.

Anthelmintics (antiparasitic herbs): Wormwood herb, neem leaf, clove bud, black walnut hulls, pomegranate fruit, pumpkin seeds.

Diagnostic questions
(these questions assess the level of risk of the digestive-regulatory type)

> Do you experience any digestive disturbances, especially bloating, abdominal fullness or congestion, or constipation?

> Do you have any symptoms that could be related to parasites— fatigue, sweet cravings, greasy stool, stomach cramps and pains, skin rashes, poor sleep, teeth-grinding, vaginal or anal itching, unexplained weight loss?

> Do you experience erratic energy levels or sugar cravings (these could be related to parasites and/or dysbiosis, not only digestive deficiency)?

Positive suggestions for the digestive-regulatory type:

▸ Your gut awareness is second to none: make your best decisions from the basis of gut instinct.

▸ Your gut is your best friend in terms of safeguarding your health: listen to it.

NOTES

1. Sharan, F. (1992). *Iridology*. London: Thorsons.
2. Gershon, M. (1998). *The Second Brain*. New York: HarperCollins.
3. Banskota, S., Ghia, J., & Khan, W. (2019). Serotonin in the gut: Blessing or a curse. *Chimie, 161*: 56–64.
4. Kriege, T., & Priest, A. (1985). *Disease Signs in the Iris*. Romford: Fowler.

5

The iris diatheses: overlay types

The third level, or facet, of the overall constitution is referred to as diathesis.

> **Diathesis, from the Greek *diatithenai*: to arrange**
>
> "A constitutional predisposition toward a particular state or condition and especially one that is abnormal or diseased." [Merriam-Webster Dictionary]

I have coined the term *overlay* for this category of appearances, since these types involve to some extent or another the presence of additional material seen in the iris that serves commonly to obscure the fiber structure. In other words, these appearances present anteriorly as you look at the iris, as a superficial build-up or overlay.

These types are especially interesting to the naturopathic practitioner because they clearly flag up the precise ways in which detoxification practices need to be applied. Detoxification is an important element of Natural Medicine therapeutics, because ridding the body of encumbrances is of vital necessity in order to facilitate the flow of vitality. I have therefore also referred to these types as the "accumulation types," since each of them points clearly to potential shortcomings in the body's clearance and elimination functions, and can pinpoint the system or systems that need to be addressed in order to resolve the build-up.

According to the research of the German iridologists Hauser, Karl, and Stolz, there are five diatheses.[1] Other writers include aspects such as the tubercular signs, or the "Central Heterochromia," but for the purposes of this book these are dealt with under "Signs and Markings." I consider there to be *four* main types.

The four main overlay types:

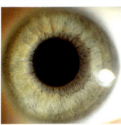

1. *Lymph rosary* (hydrogenoid diathesis)

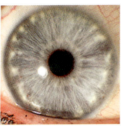

2. *Hyperacidic overlay* (hyperacidic diathesis)

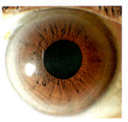

3. *Cholesterol ring* (lipemic diathesis)

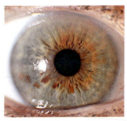

4. *Dyscratic overlay* (dyscratic diathesis)

You may have one, or more, of these types, or you may have none of them: not everyone has a diathesis, so it is important to learn to recognize the specific iris features that indicate each type. If you see one, check for the others, and if you don't see any, double check before deciding finally that there is no overlay. Where there is an identifiable overlay, application of the specific detoxification and clearance protocols outlined here will not only assist in reversing current symptoms, but will reduce future health risks preventively.

Finally, whereas constitution (color) and disposition (structure) are inherited and not expected to change, two of the four types are considered to be acquired. This means that the signs by which they are recognized are not present in younger people, typically appearing at various stages in later life. As we go through each type we will indicate where this is the case.

THE LYMPH ROSARY: HYDROGENOID DIATHESIS

The lymph rosary consists of a ring of distinct white or colored dots, sometimes in couplets, like a string of beads or pearls (hence rosary), around the outer edge of the iris. It may be complete or partial. The lymph rosary is inherited, and it can be seen in very young children. (See Figure 5.1.)

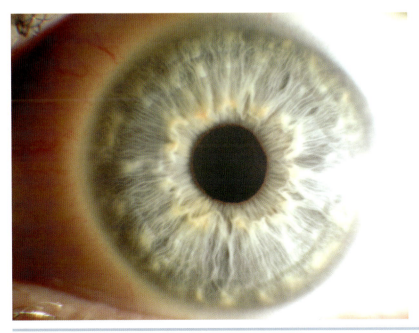

FIGURE 5.1

Lymph rosary type (hydrogenoid diathesis).

Anatomically, these dots are known as "tophi" or "Brush-field Spots" and consist of tiny bundles of fibrous material. In its complete form the lymphatic rosary is referred to as the hydrogenoid or exudative diathesis. This, again, is considered a subtype of the blue-eyed constitution; these spots also may be seen, however, in brown eyes: in the mixed iris they will bear the typical mixed coloration (Figure 5.2). I have, in fact, seen these in a hematogenic (pure dark brown) iris as well: they are difficult to pick out without either high-resolution photography or bioscopic examination, and they are generally very dark. They might appear in cases where the substance and the dense pigmentation of the iris is rarefied or thinned out in the peripheral zone; again, this might be difficult to assess in the darker iris type.

In a lymphatic iris, the spots are bright white or cream-colored. The whiteness signifies hyperreactivity and an overenthusiastic immune system. Indeed, allergy may be defined as an overactive immune response, which mounts "unnecessary" defensive reactions against ordinary, usually harmless, substances. Behind this reactivity, however, there will often be an overloading of the tissues, specifically mucous membranes and lymphatic tissue.

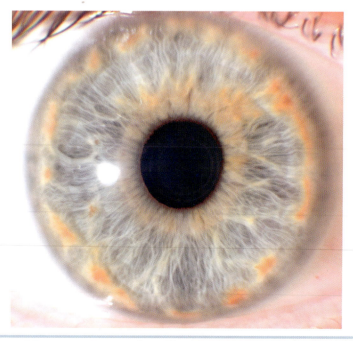

FIGURE 5.2

Hydrogenoid type with orange pigmentation of lymph tophi.

Characteristic tendencies

The word *hydrogenoid* comes from homeopathy and denotes a damp or watery constitution, and one that is also aggravated by excess moisture, especially when cold. It can be readily seen from this that it is a true subtype of the lymphatic constitution itself, and so many of the conditions and remedies discussed under the lymphatic constitution (Chapter 3) will apply to the hydrogenoid diathesis.

This sign predisposes especially to conditions affecting the upper respiratory tract, including allergic conditions like hay fever and rhinitis; phlegm and postnasal drip; tonsillitis; and swollen glands around the neck and throat. The type is also referred to as the "exudative" type: think of hay fever, especially, and you will get a sense of what this means: the constant exudation or discharge through the mucous membranes of the nasal and sinus cavities.

There is also an impact on skin, which can result in the appearance of spots, boils, and lymphatic swellings. The outer circle of the iris is associated with peripheral blood and lymph vessels and the skin, and the presence of the lymph rosary in this zone can indicate skin problems, particularly when there is also a dark outer ring—a scurf rim (see Chapter 7)—which would indicate difficulty of elimination through the skin. Lymph nodes may also be detected close to the surface, in the armpits and groin, together with skin problems such as acne or eczema.

Lymph, as noted in the discussion on the blue iris type, is all about self-cleansing and immunity. It is a clear fluid containing white blood cells whose job it is to engulf and remove debris and counteract any pathogenic influences that might threaten the integrity of the tissues; again, it is important to remember the inadvisability of suppressing natural tendencies: exudation itself may be regarded as a form of self-cleansing. It is interesting that Josef Deck also considered the origin of the sign to be rooted in a genetic or family history of tuberculosis, which is also an idea derived from homeopathy. In homeopathic terms, however, the survival of the diathesis into downline generations itself presupposes a suppression of the original disease manifestation, rather than a true cure.

Psychologically, the concern with cleaning and cleansing can translate into obsessions around tidiness and cleanliness. This usually happens when natural gifts are being thwarted or unappreciated. Hydrogenoid types make excellent homemakers, interior decorators, and landscape gardeners.

Living with a lymphatic rosary

Tendencies of the hydrogenoid type

> stifled lymph drainage leading to frequent focal infections—especially of the upper respiratory tract—e.g., tonsillitis;

> "atopic" immune reactivity (allergy)—hay fever, asthma, eczema;

> skin outbreaks and exudations—eczema, acne, boils, abscesses;

> the gut-associated lymphatic tissue (GALT), which accounts for over 50% of all lymph tissue in the body, may also be affected.

Aggravating lifestyle factors

Foods that are considered damp, or mucus-forming, will tend to aggravate the tendencies of the type, and it can be readily observed in practice that dairy produce, in particular, is not well tolerated. In addition, the "usual suspects"—sugar and refined carbohydrates—along with any undue coldness or wateriness in the diet (too much raw food or salad) will also exacerbate the natural tendencies of the type.

Exercise

The lymphatic system is part of the circulatory system, but it operates without the assistance of the heart to pump it around the body. It therefore moves only if you do, so exercise is crucial.

Exercise that works especially well for the type includes yoga, swimming, and rebounding (mini trampoline). Deep abdominal breathing also works well for people of this type, because expanding through the diaphragm causes a massaging effect on the central lymph vessel, the thoracic duct, thus helping to move the lymph around.

Hydration

Although the hydrogenoid diathesis is considered to be damp in nature, adequate water intake is also important, as lymph needs to be recycled and cleansed. Detoxification always needs to be accompanied by the replacement of old, dirty fluids with new, fresh, oxygenated fluids.

Hydrotherapy

Topical use of alternating hot and cold water (e.g., under the shower, or in saunas, steam rooms, and spas) can help power-fully to activate lymph by moving it to and from the peripheral and deep lymphatic zones. Infrared saunas are useful in that they penetrate specifically to the subcutaneous lymph tissue.

Herbal choices

Echinacea: Today known as the ultimate immune-enhancing herb, Echinacea is traditionally described as a lymph cleanser ("alterative"). Among other immune-related actions, it promotes the production of phagocytes, which are large white blood cells responsible for mopping up debris and infective material. Take a course every so often to optimize immune functions and clear the lymphatic system of congestive material. As an immunomodulator, it is also well placed to deal with allergic reactions.

Cleavers: This is a well-known spring cleanser; it also known as goose grass, bedstraw, or sticky willy. Best used as a fresh cold infusion in the Spring, when it is abundantly available in Northern European countries.

Other herbs: The following herbs can also be used, as tinctures or teas, to stimulate lymphatic cleansing and to relieve the burden on mucous membranes: mullein, nettle, burdock, calendula, bayberry, and golden seal.

Herbs to soothe mucous membranes and reduce allergic reactions are plantain (ribwort), nettle, mullein, eyebright, marsh-mallow, and licorice.

Advanced lymphatic cleansers are poke root, lobelia, and chaparral tinctures. These are not advised without professional support. It is necessary to use more gentle cleansers in preparation before taking these herbs, to avoid possible side effects.

THE HYPERACIDIC OVERLAY: HYPERACIDIC DIATHESIS

A generalized cloudiness over the iris disk indicates a tendency to accumulate metabolic acidic wastes that your body may have difficulty in eliminating. The hyperacidic overlay is inherited and can be seen in young children. It will not reduce with detoxification or alkalization. (See Figure 5.3.)

The hyperacidic type is a cloudy iris, containing wisps, clouds, and plaques in the ciliary zone (the outer part of the iris, outside the collarette). It will usually be seen in a lighter iris type, and in a blue or pale iris it will also sometimes be colored with diffuse yellow pigment, giving a greenish appearance that is sometimes referred to as the "urinary type" (Figure 5.4), and indicates that the kidneys may be under stress, particularly from incompletely digested protein residues entering the blood from a congested colon. In such a case, as well as supporting the kidneys, the bowels should be cleansed regularly in order to reduce the risk factor.

The skin, which discharges uric acid through perspiration, may also need attention. People who have clouds, wisps, and plaques in their irides hold a lot in, both physiologically and emotionally, and sometimes feel like they can't take on anything else. They need to work on letting things go emotionally. They can be resistant to therapy, since they feel that even taking this on is burdensome. The presence of a *scurf rim* (see Chapter 7) amplifies the tendencies of the hyperacidic type, and increases the tendency to hold things in.

In addition, the stomach zone itself, immediately around the pupil, frequently presents as dark and thus underactive, indicating low gastric acid production (hypochlorhydria). This compromises digestion and makes it more likely that acidic residues will arise specifically as a result of poor digestion. There is a direct

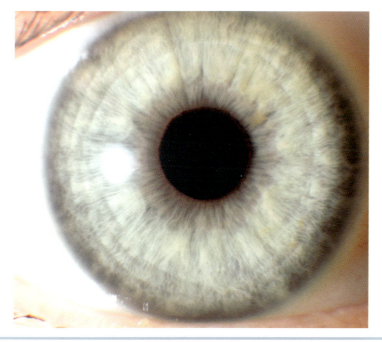

FIGURE 5.3

Hyperacidic overlay (hyperacidic diathesis).

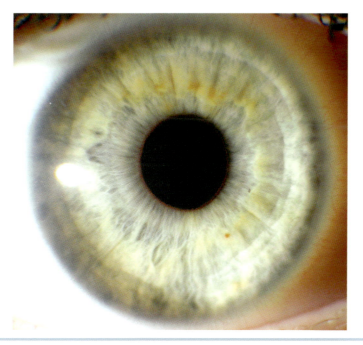

FIGURE 5.4

The "urinary" type.

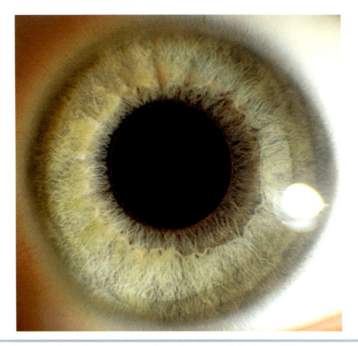

FIGURE 5.5

Hyperacidic diathesis with dark outer zone (scurf rim) and dark pupillary zone (hypochlorhydria).

correlation between high levels of acids in the tissues and in the blood, and low levels of hydrochloric acid in the stomach. (See Figure 5.5.)

The pH (potential hydrogen) "acid-base" scale ranges from 0 to 14. The readings are based around a pH of 7, which is neutral, like pure water.

> pH below 7 is acidic;

> pH higher than 7 is alkaline or *basic*.

Each level is 10 times bigger than the next. For example, a pH of 9 is 10 times more alkaline than a pH of 8. A pH of 2 is 10 times more acidic than a pH of 3, and 100 times more acidic than a reading of 4.

The pH of human blood should fall between 7.35 and 7.45. This is a fairly narrow range, which, if exceeded either way, will lead to serious illness and death. (For comparison, the pH of stomach acid should be somewhere between 1 and 3.)

Characteristic tendencies

The type shows a predisposition to metabolic acidosis, which is the abnormal retention of metabolic acidic waste material. This can arise as a result of faults in the metabolization of acids via the liver; poor food choices, and inefficient digestive processes producing higher amounts of residues; or inefficient elimination via the kidneys. It can also arise through inefficient elimination of carbon dioxide via the lungs, or through an insufficiency of neutralizing bases (alkaline buffers). Pathological causes can also include dehydration, heart failure, hypoglycemia and diabetes (diabetic acidosis), digestive problems such as vomiting and diarrhea (through fluid loss), and kidney failure.

It is important to emphasize, however, that some of these causes are also long-term pathological developments and are not necessarily predictions for the type. We have here a *risk factor* for acidosis, and, like any other iris appearance or sign, it focuses our attention on a mechanism of disease that can be avoided or reduced with the right lifestyle advice.

Robert O. Young[2] makes the long-understood naturopathic case for acidosis being a precondition of all chronic disease, including the "Big Four"—heart disease, cancer, diabetes, and autoimmune disease—the top killers in our culture. These major chronic pathologies are currently present in epidemic proportions among our populations—so much so that in the recent Covid-19 pandemic one doctor wrote to the *British Medical Journal* to suggest that technically the "pandemic" was actually a "syndemic"—it was known to kill people who were already sick, even if as yet undiagnosed, with one or more of these conditions.[3]

Very early on in my own naturopathic training I was given an "Acid–Alkaline Food Chart" as a guide to eating in such a way as to maintain optimum pH as a precondition of both prevention and cure. I now use a similar resource to give to my patients (Table 5.1). Because of the widespread consumption of acid-forming foods in our culture, I find this necessary throughout the different iris types, for reasons that should by now have started to appear obvious. Although this type is its own entity, the principle of acidic pH as a cause of chronic disease can be seen at work throughout the main constitutional types and diatheses. The link between acidosis and cardiovascular disease is mentioned in the

Table 5.1   A simple acid–alkaline food chart

Food type	Acid-forming	Alkaline-forming
Beverages	Alcohol, coffee, black tea, sugary drinks, fruit juices. Rice, oat and soy milks are mildly acidic.	High pH water (8 or above), green drinks, almond milk, coconut milk.
Animal foods	All meats, shellfish, farmed and ocean fish, eggs, dairy produce. Wild freshwater fish is only mildly acidic.	None.
Grains	Most except quinoa and buckwheat.	Quinoa, buckwheat, spelt.
Pulses	Black beans, chickpeas, kidney beans.	Lentils, tofu, butter beans, soy beans, white haricot, sprouted pulses.
Nuts & seeds	Brazil, pecan, hazel, sunflower.	Almonds, chia, flax seeds, coconut.
Fruits	Dried fruit, apple, apricot, peach, banana, grapes, mango, orange, pineapple, strawberry, berries.	Lemon, lime, avocado, tomato, grapefruit.
Vegetables	Mushrooms, potatoes (except new baby potatoes).	Most, including all leafy greens, carrot, broccoli, brussels sprouts, cauliflower, asparagus, artichoke, onion, red onion, zucchini, rhubarb, peas, swede, turnip, parsnip, new baby potatoes.
Other	Sunflower oil, grapeseed oil, artificial sweeteners and flavourings.	Most herbs and spices; avocado, olive, coconut, & flax oils; natural salt.

discussion on the hematogenic constitution, and we will see more under the lipemic diathesis (cholesterol ring) and the dyscratic diathesis. This is because the main overall outcome of acidosis, however mild, is hypoxia—low oxygen provision—which will tend to undermine health on all levels.

Please note that, in order to preserve health, the idea is not to avoid all acid-forming foods, but to keep them in strict proportion. The ideal ratio is 80/20 in favour of alkaline: most people are doing well if they get somewhere near 70/30. Of course, it does also depend on each individual's constitution.

For the purposes of most individuals sporting a hyperacidic overlay, the most likely long-term outcome of chronic failure to manage the situation is arthritic and rheumatic inflammation, including, of course, gout, which has recently been classified as an autoimmune disease, but which is commonly understood to be caused by a buildup of uric acid in the joints.

The kidneys may be at risk, as they are responsible for discharging these waste substances, so they should be specifically assessed in anyone with a hyperacidic overlay—from the point of view of iridology, this means examination of the kidney reflex zones in the irides for signs of accumulation of weakness. (On how to read signs, see Chapter 7.) There may also be a risk of kidney stones of any kind, but especially calcium oxalate and uric acid.

Psychologically, people of this type may readily declare that they "can't take any more on" and may quickly get full up and fed up, and to let those around them know!

Living with a hyperacidic overlay

Tendencies of the hyperacidic type

> ‣ formation of excess acid residues from food/digestion;
> ‣ retention of acid wastes in tissues and blood;
> ‣ hypoxia and poor cellular respiration;
> ‣ long-term drift into chronic disease, especially arthritic and rheumatic inflammation.

First and foremost, drink plenty of water to flush out and buffer the acids. Adopt an alkaline diet, rich in minerals such as calcium, magnesium, sodium, and potassium—the alkaline buffers, which will help to neutralize excess acids. The predominant items in such a diet should be *vegetables*.

Avoid red meat, pork, and pig products (all high in uric acid), excessive alcohol, coffee, and some grain foods, especially wheat. Eat plenty of fresh fruits and vegetables and drink *fresh* green juices. Chlorella is especially useful. The minimum guide for an alkaline diet is 60% fresh fruits and vegetables and 40% split between proteins, carbohydrates, and fats. In the summer the proportions can be changed to 80/20—in fact, 80/20 is considered optimal in all situations, but it may be extremely difficult to get people to sign up to this immediately. It is important to assess the baseline (most people are probably around 40% or less alkaline foods) and make what improvements you can.

Avoid and manage **stress** at all costs: it is one of the most acidifying influences out there, not least because it undermines the correct functioning of all metabolic mechanisms—kidneys, liver, digestion, immunity, nerves, and hormones—and thus impairs normal function across several parameters.

Herbal choices

Detox: The following formula, taken as part of a detox initiative, will reliably remove acidic wastes:

You will need:
- *2 parts dandelion leaf*
- *2 parts nettle herb*
- *1 part celery seed*

Use 2 heaped teaspoons of the herbs per cup of freshly boiled water; steep for at least 10 minutes, preferably 15. Do this 3 times daily during your detox. (For precise detox instructions, see Chapter 10.)

The juice of celery stalks can also be taken for this purpose.

Herbs to enhance kidney function: dandelion leaf, nettle leaf and seed, goldenrod herb, uva ursi leaf, buchu leaf, juniper berries, and asparagus root (Shatavari). Cayenne powder or tincture can

be added in small quantities as a kidney stimulant for those hardy enough to withstand the heat! (See also the kidney flush routine in Chapter 10.)

THE CHOLESTEROL RING: LIPEMIC DIATHESIS

This diathesis is identified by the presence of an opaque white circle around the outer zone of the iris. It builds up in the eye slowly over time, generally beginning as a partial ring or arc and gradually expanding to complete the ring. This diathesis is considered to be acquired—it is not seen in younger people. It is, however, likely that there is an underlying genetic or familial influence. (See Figure 5.6.)

The word "lipemic" means "relating to blood fats." This medically recognized sign is also called the *lipemic annulus* ("blood fat ring"), the sodium ring, or the *arcus senilis* ("the arc of old age").

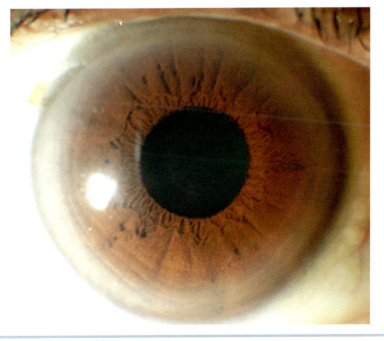

FIGURE 5.6

The "cholesterol ring" (lipemic diathesis)

The sign actually appears as a result of a buildup of material in the cornea, not the iris, although it obscures the outer ring of the iris as you look at it. It is a sign for the tendency to develop high blood fats and atherosclerosis—"plaquing" of the arteries, with the concomitant risk of ischemic circulatory disease—and narrowing of critical blood vessels supplying blood to the heart, the brain, or the lower extremities.

Bernard Jensen,[4] who called it the "sodium ring," refers to it in terms of minerals "out of solution"—that is, deposited on the inside of arteries. This also refers to the fact that arterial plaques are made of more than just cholesterol: they have a complex consistency that may also include minerals, especially calcium, which is responsible for the term "hardening of the arteries."

Although it is a medically recognized sign for the presence of high blood fats (including cholesterol), many doctors also consider it a natural sign of old age. When it appears in the upper segment of the iris, it is referred to as the *arcus senilis* (arc of old age) and portends possible memory problems or, at its most extreme, a stroke or senile dementia (Figure 5.7). It indicates insufficient nourishment and oxygenation of the cerebral circulation, leading to poor function of the brain. The fully developed ring, or annulus, also

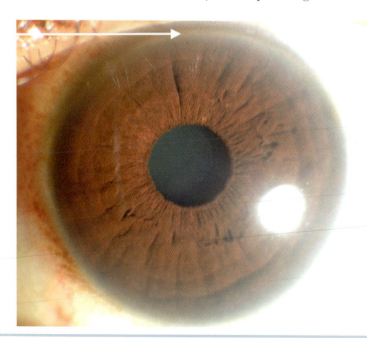

FIGURE 5.7

The frontal arcus, or "arcus senilis."

warns of possible coronary arterial blockage, leading to myocardial infarction—death of part of the heart muscle, or a heart attack; or, if found predominantly in the lower sector of the irides, compromise to the lower extremities, leading to peripheral arterial disease.

It is much more common in people with pure dark brown irides (hematogenic) than in the other two constitutional types; it can, however, occur in all types (see Figures 5.8 and 5.9). Because it is not a sign seen from birth, it is assumed to be evidence of an *acquired* condition. However, although it only appears as life progresses, it is very often seen in cases of so-called "familial" high cholesterol and so is also considered to portray a genetic predisposition to difficulty with regulating blood fats. It can begin to appear as early as the mid-20s (in hematogenic types) but is more usually first seen as a faint, translucent hazy ring between the ages of 40 and 50; if nothing is done to reverse it, it will continue to develop.

The iris sign is peculiar by virtue of two apparently paradoxical findings: on the one hand, the sign may be relatively advanced in the iris, but when checked, serum cholesterol levels appear normal; on the other hand, some individuals with even quite advanced disease may not display the iris sign. This, however, is a small percentage of cases. In general, I would estimate that the sign is around 85% accurate as a predictive sign for high cholesterol, and where this is found to be the case, further investigation is warranted.

The specific investigations required may, however, be the subject of some disagreement between physicians of differing approaches. From the naturopathic perspective, the "problem" is rarely cholesterol itself, but whatever is causing it to stick to the sides. This is a highly complex phenomenon, but, as previously suggested, it has a lot to do with systemic levels of inflammation. Even when it comes to the balance of "good" vs. "bad" cholesterol, the issue is not as simple as this tends to suggest. "Bad" cholesterol—or low-density lipoprotein (LDL) cholesterol—is certainly implicated in arterial plaquing, but it is less clear what exact role it plays in the complex etiology of that condition—whether pathological, or perhaps part of a protective mechanism that seeks to provide a temporary fix to a developing problem, pending restoration to full functional normality—always the desired end result of inflammation—of the acute kind, at least.

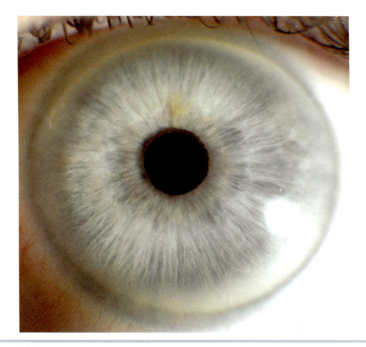

FIGURE 5.8

Lymphatic lipemic iris.

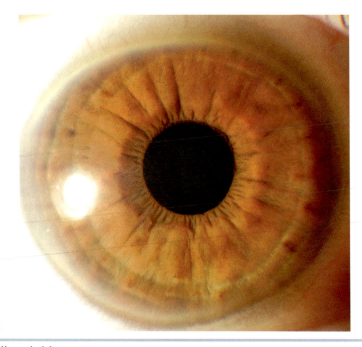

FIGURE 5.9

Mixed biliary lipemic iris.

Add to that the previously cited fact that cholesterol itself has distinct health-preserving functions (it is required for cellular repair as an integral component of cell walls, and it forms the starting material for the manufacture of hormones necessary to the stress response), as even LDL cholesterol has been found to be protective against dementia, including Alzheimer's disease, in older people.

My own, relatively simple, answer to this is to recommend a test for homocysteine, which is now (in nonmainstream circles) regarded as a more accurate assessment of actual cardiovascular risk, high levels in the blood being associated with higher risk factors in terms of ischemic circulatory disease. You can buy a home-test kit for homocysteine online.

Characteristic tendencies

Since cholesterol buildup, both in the irides and in the vessels, takes place slowly over years and even decades, there are few specific early warning symptoms, although cold extremities, particularly the feet, and failing memory, while they can be due to other causes, can sometimes be useful indicators.

Other clues affecting the digestive system may be found. Often there is a growing intolerance of rich, fatty foods. While only 15% of serum cholesterol is derived from foods (and then only from animal foods—cholesterol is an animal product, it is not found in plants), that leaves a whopping 85% potentially being manufactured "in house." Nonetheless, as the situation progresses, the liver, especially, may begin to struggle with the increased metabolic load, and symptoms may start to appear in the form of indigestion, epigastric bloating, and GERD.

Psychologically, people with this sign may appear quite stubborn, resistant to change, and set in their ways. However, they may also be described as idealistic and determined, and their resistance seen as a reluctance to have their ideals and beliefs challenged or diluted in any way. They make good campaigners for any cause. Emotionally they need to guard against a tendency to be dogmatic or overidentified with their own opinions—rigidity of thought being potentially an analogue of the rigidity that manifests in the arteries themselves.

Living with a lipemic diathesis

Tendencies of the lipemic type

> slow development of arterial deposits, considered to be caused by high levels of blood cholesterol;

> the onset of cardiovascular disease, including high blood pressure and narrowing of arteries, leading to strokes, angina, heart attacks, and other cardiovascular problems;

> digestive fullness, GERD, epigastric bloating, and weight gain;

> cold extremities, memory problems, peripheral circulatory incompetence.

In terms of the naturopathic etiology of the condition, it is to the liver that we would address much of our attention, while, of course, protecting and strengthening the heart and circulation.

A liver-friendly diet is mainly plant-based, dairy free in particular, and very high in fresh, antioxidant-rich foods, such as dark green leafy vegetables and brightly colored fruits. Vegetables with a high sulfur content, such as the onion family, including garlic and leeks, and the cabbage family, strongly support liver detoxification. Adequate hydration is crucial, and the routine addition of fresh lemon and/or lime to water is much to be encouraged—these fruits being especially cleansing to the liver.

The liver flush routine should be performed three or four times annually (see Chapter 10).

Herbal choices

Garlic, artichoke leaf, and motherwort help to protect the heart and may lower cholesterol. Remember, in this context, the old Chinese saying about the bitter flavor "entering the heart": all bitters are extremely protective in this scenario.

Hawthorn strengthens circulatory vessels and protects the heart; cayenne and ginger stimulate circulation; and ginkgo and red clover thin the blood. These herbs should be taken as teas or tinctures, with the exception of garlic, which should be eaten raw, preferably as a food.

THE DYSCRATIC OVERLAY: DYSCRATIC DIATHESIS

This type is identified by the presence of multiple secondary pigments of different colors and hues, and frequently overlapping each other. It usually occurs in a lighter iris type—frequently lymphatic, but occasionally mixed biliary. This type is considered to be acquired—it is not seen in very young people. (See Figure 5.10.)

The term *dyscratic* comes from ancient Greco–Roman humoral medicine. In this understanding the humors, or "deep body fluids," occur in each individual in an ideal mix or proportion. This was known, in those days, as *eucrasia*, which means "good mixture." Dyscrasia means the opposite: "bad mixture." A bad mixture of fluids, or humors, predisposes to disease. The term survived for a while in standard medicine to indicate intoxication or disturbance of the blood.

The appearance of dyscratic pigmentation suggests the accumulation of toxic influences affecting the system but begs the question why some people acquire this appearance and not others? Once again, it seems that there must be an underlying genetic or

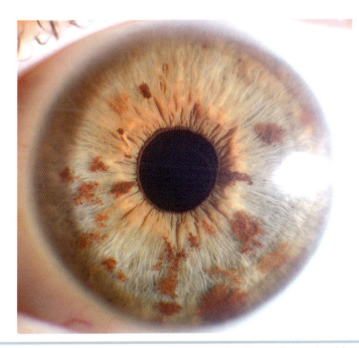

FIGURE 5.10

The dyscratic overlay (dyscratic diathesis).

inherited element, despite the fact that the signs do not generally appear in the very young.

The specific pigmentation referred to here has no relation to the primary pigmentation of the constitutional type. These pigments are called secondary and may appear in a variety of colors, ranging from pale yellow through the yellow–orange–red–brown spectrum, all the way to almost black (tar pigments). (For a full discussion of each of these colors, see the "Pigment Differentiation Chart", Table 7.1.)

These pigments are also generally not visible in the darker iris types—although they may, indeed, be present. As a comment on this, when Josef Deck first classified the iris types, his original designation for the dark brown type was *dyscratic*. He later revised this to *hematogenic*. The implication, however, is that the dyscratic diathesis replicates many of the concerns of the hematogenic constitution in the lighter iris color types.

I have personally observed this overlay, and secondary pigmentation in general, to arrive in the irides during adolescence—the growing into adulthood, in other words, between the ages of 13 and 18 (see Figure 5.10). In this approximately 5-year window many changes take place, including natural genetic regulatory and formative developments and the specific existential stresses and strains of "coming of age." Remember the story of Nils Liljequist (Chapter 1), who observed such changes in his own eyes at around that same age. Liljequist ascribed his iris changes to the administration of drugs, but what if there were another reason? The concept of genetics did not exist at the time, so perhaps his assumptions were entirely natural—and actually they have not yet been proven wrong. We must conclude that the jury is still out as to the origin of this phenomenon, but, like all other iris phenomena, it is highly likely to have a genetic basis.

Characteristic tendencies

The key understanding of the type is couched in terms of enzyme provision. If you look at the "Pigment Differentiation Chart" (Table 7.1), you will see that each color relates to a specific organ and metabolic tendency. Often this is related to the secretion of enzymes, for digestion, but also for other metabolic conver-

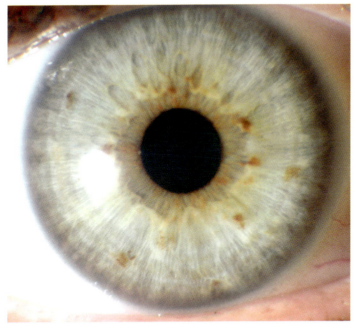

FIGURE 5.11

Lymphatic dyscratic iris,

sion and breakdown purposes. The suggestion here is that we are looking at a type in which enzyme provision may be suboptimal. (I suggest that at this point you skip forward and take a look at this chart, to provide further illustration of the principles of this discussion.)

Enzymes perform a myriad functions within our systems: they are defined as substances that act as catalysts of chemical reactions in the body without being changed by those reactions. Accordingly, they can be used over and over again. Enzymes also speed up the rate of reactions, permitting hundreds or even thousands more simultaneous operations than would be possible otherwise without taking far longer to accomplish. Examples range from the breakdown of foods in the digestive tract, through the breakdown of toxins in the liver, to the management of blood pressure and other vital homeostatic functions.

In particular it is the role of enzymes in detoxification that present themselves for consideration in this type, although it should also be noted that, as we have seen, digestive function in particular is a key element in maintaining a toxin-free system.

According to the German researchers Hauser, Karl, and Stolz, this diathesis predisposes to liver, gallbladder, and pancreatic disease (including diabetes), inflammatory joint and connective tissue diseases (soft-tissue rheumatic complaints), and cancer. It is worth noting in this connection that the link between enzyme deficiency and cancer is a lynchpin of naturopathic approaches to cancer, where high-strength enzyme supplementation is routinely applied in treatment.

A point of frequent confusion arises at the intersection of the dyscratic type and the hyperacidic type. You should be able to see in the illustration that a cloudy hyperacidic overlay is present as part of the dyscratic component: in my opinion, therefore—other researchers may have their own opinions—a strong hyperacidic tendency may be automatically assumed in the case of a dyscratic overlay. Comparing the tendencies discussed here with comments made in the section on the hyperacidic overlay, the connection is clearly evident.

Living with a dyscratic overlay

Tendencies of the dyscratic type

‣ pigments may develop in adolescent years or later;

‣ shortfall of enzyme secretion, especially for digestion and detoxi-fication;

‣ toxemia and tissue encumbrance developing over time into serious pathology: diabetes, inflammatory complaints, and even, possibly, tumor development.

Although the tendencies above may seem to be pretty frightening, we must remember that the usual rules of iridology still apply: nothing is set in stone in the iris. The iris signs are still to be regarded as our best guide to prevention *and* cure. As long as we follow the suggestions that the iris gives us, we will always have the possibility of regaining health and vitality, even when it seems quite lost.

The basic rules here are utterly simple: keep the system absolutely as clean as possible, by means of regular *deep* detoxi-

6

The iris chart

The iris chart breaks down the small disk of the iris into zones that give finely tuned information about the organs that fall within the zones. It is important to grasp the basic principles of iridology before you try to diagnose problems with individual organs or specific diseases. While studying the iris chart, it is useful to have on hand a medical dictionary and a book on anatomy. When looking at your own eyes, you can observe the presence of signs and their positions and begin to ask yourself relevant questions. Wait until you have read Chapters 7 and 8, however, before forming opinions about any problems you may have. Reading the chart is not the same as conducting a full assessment. Also, bear in mind that when you look at your own eyes in a mirror, you are seeing a reverse image and need to calculate the correct positions.

It is as well to have some familiarity with the iris chart ahead of learning about the various signs and markings that we can find in the irides: that way, once you start looking at those markings (Chapter 7), you will already be able to place them in some kind of context.

THE CONCENTRIC ZONES OF THE IRIS

The concentric zones of the iris begin at the pupil and end with the outer circle, where the iris joins the sclera, or the white of the eye (Figure 6.1).

The concentric zones act as a "metabolic flow chart," describing our tendencies in the ways absorb, digest, distribute, and utilize energy (food). It also reveals our ability to eliminate unused or toxic elements. The flow works from the center (pupil) outward.

The rings of the iris are principally divided into two zones—the collarette, or pupillary zone, and the ciliary zone (anything outside the border of the collarette). Each of these zones is then further subdivided.

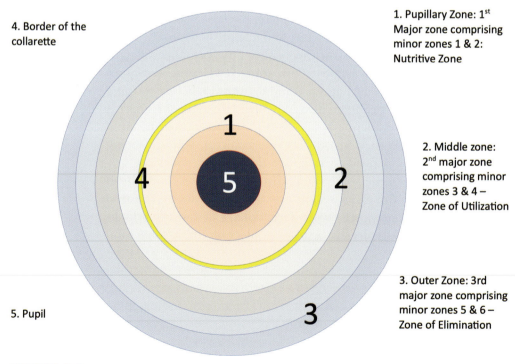

4. Border of the collarette

1. Pupillary Zone: 1st Major zone comprising minor zones 1 & 2: Nutritive Zone

2. Middle zone: 2nd major zone comprising minor zones 3 & 4 – Zone of Utilization

3. Outer Zone: 3rd major zone comprising minor zones 5 & 6 – Zone of Elimination

5. Pupil

FIGURE 6.1

Concentric zones of the iris chart.

The pupil

Actually a gap or *lumen*, you can think of the pupil as the mysterious essence of a person. As shown in Chapter 2, pupil size can give information about the autonomic nerve settings: large pupil = sympathetic dominance, small pupil = parasympathetic dominance.

The pupillary ruff

The thin red–brown ring found at the inner margin of the iris, lining the pupil, is also known as the *inner pupil border* (IPB), and the *ring of absorption*. It is the first point of contact of the pupil with physical reality and describes how we react to and digest our experiences. This structure is minute: you have to look hard to see it with a magnifier. It appears as an orange or red–brown ruff bordering the inner edge of the iris. (For a discussion of its anatomy, see Chapter 2.)

- ▶ A *thick pupillary ruff* reflects a person who greets the challenges of life with enthusiasm, possibly even aggression, and who is outwardly focused in the physical world, but who may lack appreciation for the subtler, finer energies (Figure 6.2).
- ▶ A *thin pupillary ruff* indicates a person who shies away from life's challenges and may be quite timid. This person may find the harshness of the physical world overwhelming and can be hypersensitive (Figure 6.3).

It is normal for the pupillary ruff to be of varying thickness, usually split between thicker and thinner sections on a slightly diagonal, longitudinal axis, and also to be subject to individual irregularities around its circumference. A specialist can read these irregularities and gain information about the central nervous system and how it is influenced by possible stresses on the spine. It is possible to pinpoint the exact vertebrae involved and make a diagnosis about the nerve supply to the organs indicated.

In addition, the shape of the pupil itself can give valuable information about patterns of tension and misalignment affecting the spine, such as scoliosis (Figure 6.4).

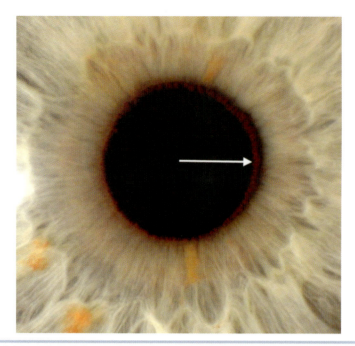

FIGURE 6.2

Thick (hypertonic) inner pupil border.

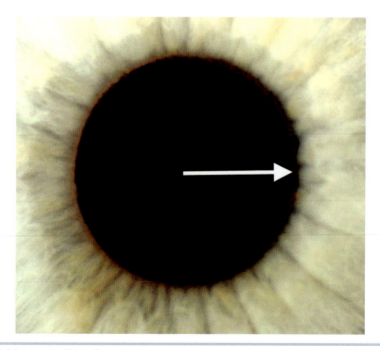

FIGURE 6.3

Thin (hypotonic) inner pupil border.

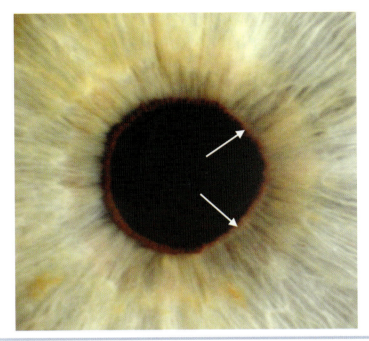

FIGURE 6.4

Close-up showing flattened sections of the pupil circumference.

THREE MAJOR ZONES/SIX MINOR ZONES OF THE IRIS

First major zone: stomach and intestinal rings

This is also known as the *pupillary* or *nutritive zone.*

Stomach ring

The next circular zone after the pupillary ruff can sometimes be seen as a regular, whitish (in a pale eye) halo just around the pupil (Figure 6.5). It generally reflects the position of the sphincter muscle, which lies beneath it in the iris body, and it can be seen clearly in some blue or pale mixed eyes.

The color and shading of the stomach ring is significant. Bright whiteness suggests overreactivity: in this case, the tendency to produce too much hydrochloric acid and a disposition to

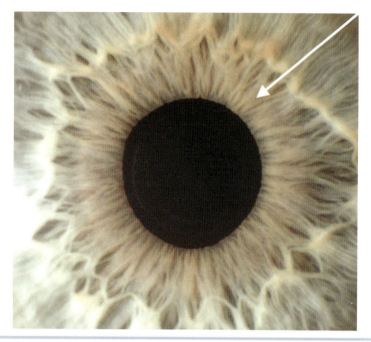

FIGURE 6.5

Close-up showing position of the stomach halo.

gastritis and gastric ulcers. A gray or muddy-looking stomach ring is an indication of a sluggish supply of digestive secretions from the stomach, and consequent failure to digest food properly. A normal stomach ring is not too dark, not too bright. Don't worry if you can't see yours. It is usually not visible in brown eyes and is not visible in all blue eyes.

The *stomach ring* is also designated the *first minor zone*.

Intestinal ring

Still within the pupillary zone, and the first major zone, the area immediately around the stomach ring is known as the *intestinal ring*. It is contained and given shape on the other side by the border of the collarette, which typically takes a varied course and is rarely perfectly circular (Figure 6.6).

The ins and outs of the border of the collarette graphically describe the condition of the intestines. Areas of distension can indicate constipation, and an environment in which toxic and degenerative conditions are able to take hold (see "The Digestive-

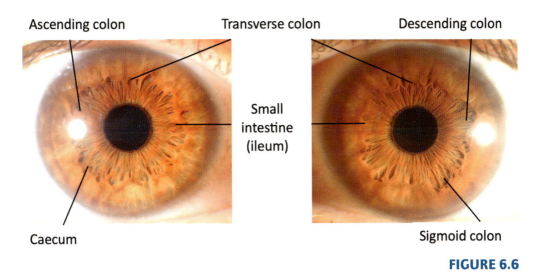

Ascending colon   Transverse colon   Descending colon

Small
intestine
(ileum)

Caecum   Sigmoid colon

FIGURE 6.6

Intestinal reflex areas in the irides.

Regulatory Iris," in Chapter 4). Conversely, where the collarette border draws in, there can be strictures or spasmodic conditions affecting the intestines. The collarette may also be partially expanded, where it seems to invade the space of another organ. This can indicate consequences for that organ, which may be under pressure—for example, from congestion or other suboptimal conditions in the bowel. The intestinal ring also includes the sections of the small intestine (see "Signs Affecting the Border of the Collarette," in Chapter 7).

The *intestinal ring* is also designated the *second minor zone*.

Second major zone:
utilization and ultimate utilization

The second major zone makes up what is referred to as the "mid-ciliary" area. (The ciliary zone is so-named because behind the iris in this location is a circular nerve plexus known as the "ciliary body"). It extends from the collarette border to approximately two thirds the way out toward the iris edge and is similarly divided, into the third and the fourth minor zones.

The humoral zone

Just outside the border of the collarette is a thin band referred to separately as the humoral zone. It is the location of many of the endocrine organ reflex fields (Figure 6.7). (See "The Hormone-Regulatory Iris," in Chapter 4.)

Also known as the "zone of distribution and transportation," its position just outside the digestive reflexes gives it special signifi-

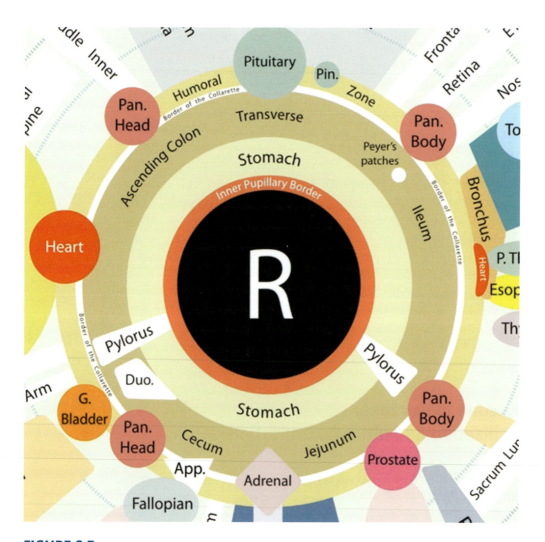

FIGURE 6.7

Close-up of iris chart showing detail of digestive and humoral zones (the first, second,

cance for the way food is taken up and transported by the blood vessels surrounding the small intestine, and for the portal system— the blood flow into the liver and spleen, which is essential for processing nutriment.

Jensen's iris chart gives the letters "MES" in this position, standing for "mesentery." The mesentery consists of a web of connective tissue that attaches the intestines to the poste- rior abdominal wall and is formed by a double fold of the

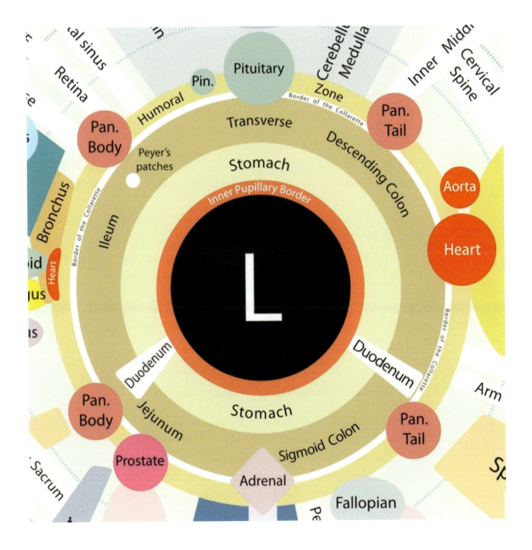

and third minor zones).

peritoneum—the sheath containing and protecting the abdominal organs. Its function is to connect all parts of the intestinal tract to a blood supply, lymphatic vessels, and nerves—the "essential services"—but it is into the blood supply carried by this structure that food particles broken down in the digestive tract are first absorbed for onward transportation: first to the liver (via the portal system) for the "first pass" safety check (detoxification), and then made available to the whole system.

There may be implications, too, for gastrointestinal immunity, as there is a large amount of lymph tissue located around the gastrointestinal organs. Any area of the body open to outside influences, as the digestive tract is, must be defended against potential disease-causing organisms. The immune system regards anything entering the body as potentially harmful and monitors it all.

Lymph tissue is, incidentally, present also in specific aggregations throughout the digestive tract—in the throat and the upper respiratory tract (tonsils, adenoids), the small intestine (Peyer's patches), and at the beginning of the colon, the caecum (the appendix).

The humoral zone is therefore an extremely important zone to monitor. Congestive appearances, specifically, may imply impediments to the absorption and distribution of nutriments, overloading of the deep-level circulatory vessels, and, of course, hormonal disruptions and irregularities, while the presence of lacunae in this concentric location gives rise to the hormone-regulatory iris disposition, as has already been discussed. (See Figure 6.8.)

Third minor zone: zone of utilization

This zone, taking in the humoral zone at its inner margin, concerns the body's use of nutriment. Here we find most of the major organs outside the digestive tract—for example, the liver, kidneys, bladder, spleen, brain, and lungs. These are the organs that take up the energy from food and use it to keep us going. Having ingested, broken down, and distributed food, the body now puts it to work. Interruptions or congestive appearances in this field suggest a poor movement of nutritional and vital energy through these organs. (See Figure 6.9.)

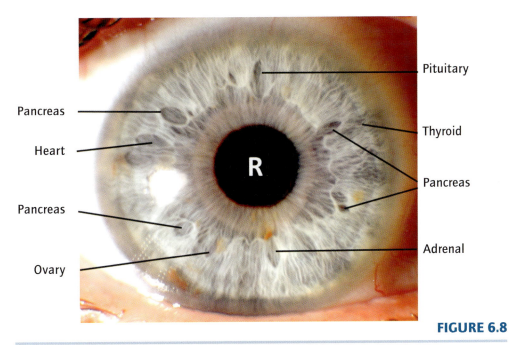

Pituitary

Pancreas

Heart

Thyroid

Pancreas

Pancreas

Ovary

Adrenal

FIGURE 6.8

Positions of hormonal organs in the humoral zone.

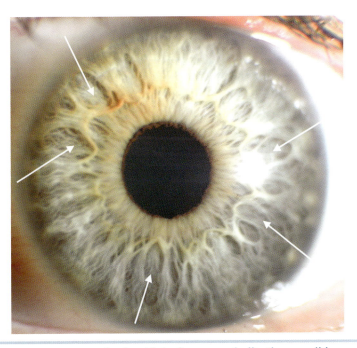

FIGURE 6.9

Lacunae in the third minor zone, indicating possible organ weaknesses.

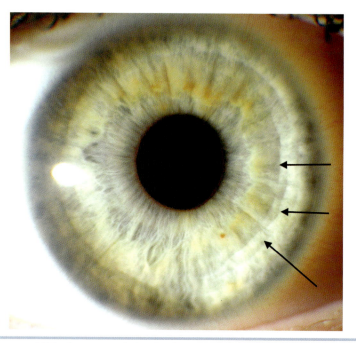

FIGURE 6.10

White cloudy (hyperacidic) plaques and circular (tension) furrows in the fourth minor zone: predisposition to arthritis.

Fourth minor zone: zone of ultimate utilization

This zone specifically contains the musculoskeletal system. The skeleton is also a store of minerals—especially calcium—for future use. Signs of weakness can indicate a tendency to mineral deficiency, possibly osteoporosis. White, inflammatory, or congestive signs in this band may indicate arthritic or rheumatic disease. (See Figure 6.10.)

Third major zone: the outer zone or zone of elimination

Starting approximately two thirds of the way out from the border of the collarette toward the outer edge of the iris, this zone is similarly divided into two minor zones, the fifth and sixth: the *lymphatic zone*, and the *skin zone*

Fifth minor zone: peripheral lymph and circulation

This is the zone in which the lymph rosary appears (Figure 6.11). (See Chapter 5.)

Sixth minor zone: skin and products of skin (integument)

Known especially when dark shading is present as the "scurf rim," which may indicate underactivity of the skin but also skin problems, such as eczema (see Chapter 7). It also suggests a closed-down periphery, possibly adaptive in the sense of conserving heat, but bringing its own problems in terms of reduced perspiration and therefore less elimination of acidic wastes (Figure 6.12). (See also "The Hyperacidic Overlay," in Chapter 5.)

The limbus or iris root

At the very outer edge of the iris we find the limbus, where the iris is joined to the sclera. There are also a range of "ring sign" appearances that can give useful data located at this concentric position. (See "Ring Signs," in Chapter 7.)

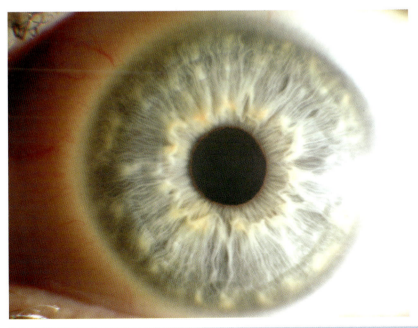

FIGURE 6.11

The lymph rosary in the fifth minor zone.

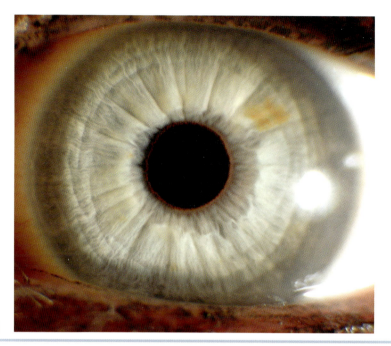

FIGURE 6.12

Dark outer band (scurf rim) in the sixth minor zone.

THE IRIS REFLEX CHART: RADIAL POSITIONS

The concept that one part of the body contains clues about the rest of the system is not unique to iridology. Reflexology and Chinese face reading are two other well-known systems, both of which include a reflex pattern, in which the feet and the hands or the face contain allotted points relating to all the other organs of the body.

The first iris chart, produced by Ignácz von Péczely in the mid-nineteenth century, forms the basis upon which most charts are drawn up. Von Péczely's chart has many of the organs in the same places that iridologists still recognize today (see chapter 1).

Over the years, many different iris charts have been created. Most of these agree on the basic positions, with differences mainly in the amount of detail shown.

The German iridologist and naturopath, Joseph Angerer,[1] produced one of the most detailed charts. His research led him to break down the iris into smaller reflex zones that give very finely detailed information about the organs and their individual parts. However, without close microscopy it can be difficult to match the minutiae of such a chart to the actual iris, so most iridologists choose something a little less detailed. One of the most influential and well-known charts is Bernard Jensen's, and many modern charts have been developed from his.

The chart presented here (Figure 6.13) has been drawn up to reflect the major current agreed positions in iris topography, while at the same time remaining simple and readable, not overcrowded, and yet with enough detail to enable a precise reading.

WORKING WITH THE IRIS REFLEX CHART

How to look at the chart

You can look at it from the front, as though you are facing the body, or from the top down—that is, through the central lumen of the human body, as if you are traveling through the gastrointestinal tract. Taking the view from the front, you can see some basic correspondences: the brain is at the top, the lungs on each side, the liver mainly on the right, the spleen on the left, and the heart mainly on the left, but with a reflex site on the right, too. Some of these observations reflect the embryological development of the body.

When looking at the chart, remember that it is drawn up as if you are facing the individual, so the left eye will be to your right. The convention is to use positions of the clock, rather than degrees, to locate the organs: top dead center of the iris is 12 o'clock or 0 minutes, the opposite is 6 o'clock or 30 minutes.

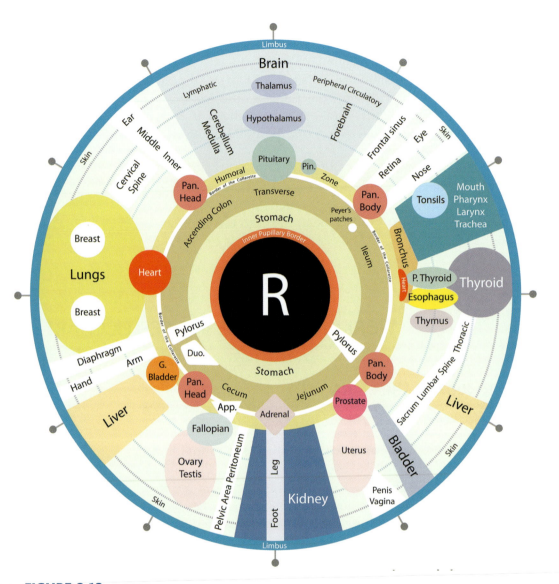

FIGURE 6.13

Chart of iris topography. (The College of Holistic Iridology; Copyright 2023.)

App. = appendix.   Duo. = duodenum.

Pan. Head = head of pancreas.   Pan. Body = pancreas body.   Pan. Tail = pancreas tail.

Pin. = pineal gland.   P. Thyroid = parathyroid.

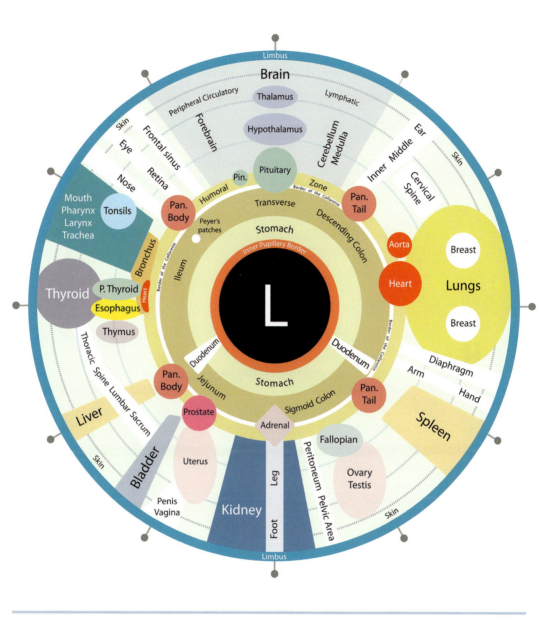

The brain

Located between 55 minutes and 05 minutes in the left and right irides, the brain can be subdivided into areas reflecting the different parts. Note the position of the pituitary gland and, above it, the hypothalamus and the thalamus (Figure 6.14). (The "master" hormone gland, the pituitary, is discussed under "The Hormone-Regulatory Iris," Chapter 4.)

The hypothalamus, linked to the pituitary below and the thalamus above, controls body temperature, hunger and thirst, sleep, balance, sexual function, and emotional function. It also has links to both the hormonal and autonomic nervous systems through its control of pituitary secretions.

The thalami (there is one in each hemisphere of the brain) are thought to be the seats of conscious awareness of physical

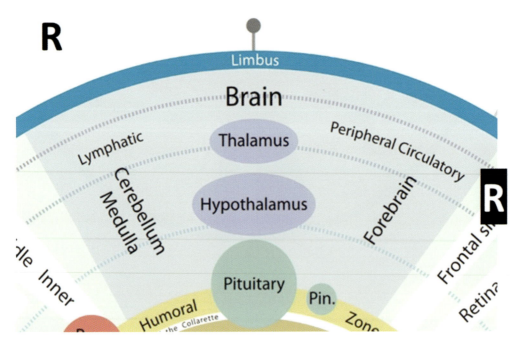

FIGURE 6.14

Close-up of brain reflex areas in the iris chart.

stimuli and act as relay stations to transmit these to the lower centers. They also feed into the hypothalamus—hence, sensations received by the thalamus closely affect the functions of this center and also of the pituitary.

Note also the position of the pineal gland at 3 minutes (right iris) and 57 minutes (left iris). This gland is involved in the secretion of the "sleep hormone," melatonin, among several other hormones having various correspondences—for example, to sexual function; when aspected—having, for example, a crypt on that position in either iris—there can be sleep disturbances.

However, one of the main functions of the pineal gland is in the absorption and transmission of light as energy throughout the system. In esoteric traditions the pineal gland serves as the third eye, or spiritual sight. Signs affecting the pineal gland may also be checked out for links to depression and melancholy, and for

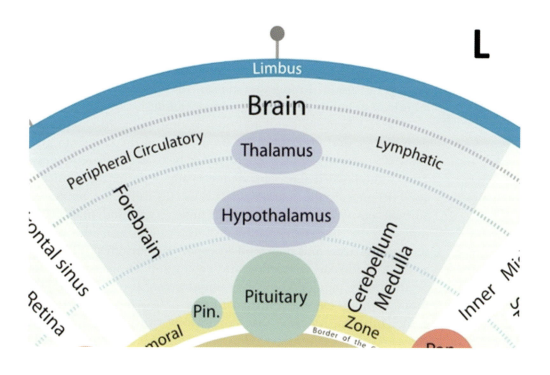

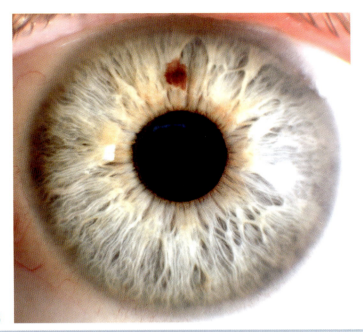

FIGURE 6.15

In this iris a large lacuna and a pigment are seen coinciding in the pituitary-hypothalamus location.

seasonal affective disorder (SAD syndrome), where the individual suffers low mood during the shorter, darker days of the winter months, essentially through light deprivation.

The link between mind and body is close to the heart of holistic iridology, and observation of these areas on the chart can give clues as to how susceptible a person may be to stress-related illness. This is amplified if the point diametrically opposite the pituitary, at 30 minutes, is also marked. This is usually called the pituitary/adrenal axis. When marked with lacunae, crypts, indentations of the collarette, or radial furrows, it indicates a person who is very sensitive to stress and may tend to experience health problems as a result, particularly depletion and exhaustion. However, a lacuna or secondary pigmentation at 0 minutes can also reflect opportunities for developing spiritual insight or psychic abilities. This is the zone that relates to our connection with higher regions of consciousness. (The subject shown in Figure 6.15 was experiencing chronic fatigue as a result of years of work stress. A radical change in life direction was indicated.)

The digestive system

You are now familiar with the arrangement of the gastrointestinal tract around the pupil. You will see that there are some specific areas that relate to different parts of the stomach, duodenum, jejunum, small intestine, and ascending, transverse, and descending sections of the colon. Regarding the latter, you can trace the ascending colon from the right eye, the transverse from the right to left eye, and the descending colon down through the left eye, reflecting the peristaltic flow in the colon. (See Figure 6.16.)

Note the junction of the thin slice that describes the esophagus at 45 minutes in the left eye and 15 minutes in the right, with the central ring of the nutritive zone. At this point, a weakness marking could indicate the possibility of a hiatus hernia or weakness of the lower esophageal sphincter (LOS). (See "The Mixed Biliary Constitution," in Chapter 3.) However, note also that this position coincides and overlaps with one of the heart reflexes—that's why gastroesophageal reflux disease (GERD) is popularly known as *heartburn*—and is often mistaken for a cardiac pathology. (In a case of an iris like the one shown in Figure 6.17, check for GERD, but also for cardiac symptoms.)

In addition to the digestive tract itself, there are some other organs that need to be assessed as part of the digestive system. These are the liver, gallbladder, pancreas, and the spleen.

The liver, gallbladder, spleen, and pancreas

The liver is located in the right iris at 37 to 40 minutes and 22 minutes, and in the left iris at 37 minutes. The gallbladder is at 40 minutes in the right iris, close to the collarette. The spleen is located in the left iris at 20–22 minutes.

The sectors at approximately 20 and 40 minutes in each eye are the liver and spleen reflexes. The liver, being a very large organ, accounts for three of these sites. The liver is situated mainly on the right side of the body; however, the left lobe crosses the median line, so we get a sublocation of the liver in the left iris at 37 minutes.

Assessment of these zones is frequently advised, as the liver does an immense amount of work and can become congested and inflamed. When treated correctly, it regenerates extremely well, so

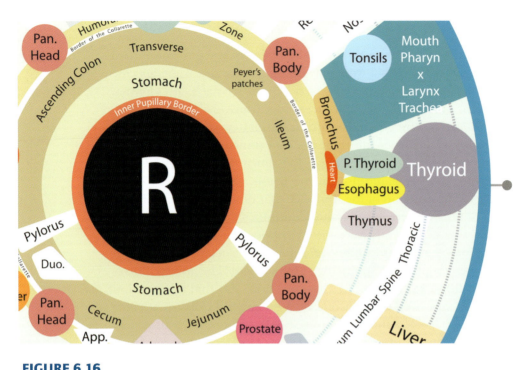

FIGURE 6.16

Section showing reflex positions for the different areas of the digestive tract.

it pays to cleanse and tone it and its many functions from time to time. (For instructions on how to make the liver-flush drink, see Chapter 10.)

There are several pigment appearances that are described as *hepatotropic*—that is, they indicate liver involvement. These do not necessarily appear directly on liver reflex zones but may be found anywhere; this is the "principle of topolability" (see Chapter 7). However, always check the liver reflexes on the chart. Signs of deficiency—lacunae or thinning of iris tissue—may indicate underfunctioning, and this can have repercussions on digestion, detoxification, and hormone function. White signs and pigment signs may reveal inflammatory and congestive tendencies. Note in Figure 6.18 the cluster of extra-white fibers in the main liver reflex, as well as the transversal fibers (running "across the grain") in both liver positions, indicating possible irritation/inflammation in the liver. (See Figure 6.18.)

Note the cluster of extra-white fibers in the main liver reflex

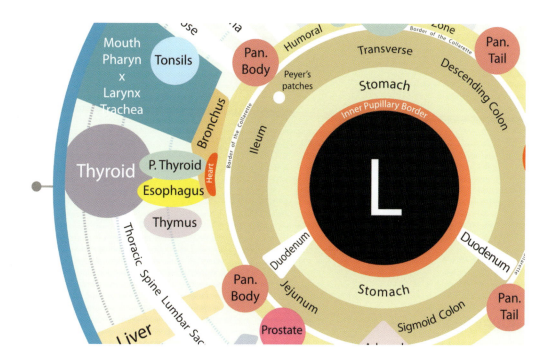

in this right eye; also transversal fibers (running "across the grain") in both liver positions: possible irritation/inflammation in the liver.

The spleen: There is a discussion to be had here about the spleen. The iris reflex site between 20 and 22 minutes in the left iris refers to the Western anatomical spleen, which is part of the vascular system and the immune system. When aspected by, for example, lacunae or thinning of iris tissue (rarefaction), there can be weak or suppressed immunity (Figure 6.19).

However it is also the case that the Chinese organ, the spleen, which refers to the overall function of digestion in supplying nutriment to the entire organism, may also be checked in these locations. It would not be fully accurate to equate the pancreas with the TCM spleen, as there is much more involved (many functions of the spleen are well described by the term "transportation and distribution," for example, which would be mapped in the humoral zone—see above): however, many people agree that

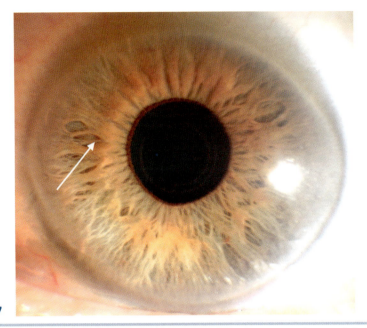

FIGURE 6.17

Lacuna impinging on the junction of esophagus with collarette at 45 minutes, left iris.

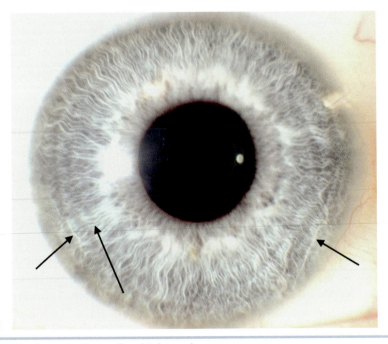

FIGURE 6.18

Extra-white fibers in the main liver reflex (right eye)
and transversal fibers in both liver positions.

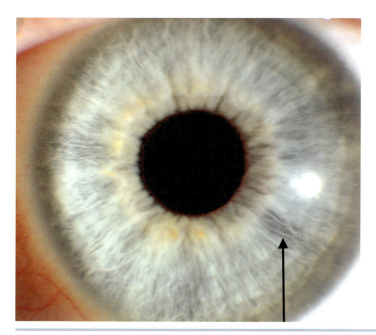

FIGURE 6.19

Rarefaction (thinning of iris tissue) in the location of the spleen reflex: possible compromised immunity.

weak or compromised pancreatic function will have a very similar outcome to that which would be expected from TCM "spleen qi deficiency": poor digestion, pale stools, accumulation of damp, and possible long-term development of diabetes.

The pancreas: The function of the pancreas, like the liver, has far-reaching effects upon the whole system, yet few people even know where it is and what it does. It is set on the left side of the upper abdomen, behind the stomach. It secretes pancreatic juices, rich in enzymes, for the breakdown of foods—particularly of carbohydrates.

On the iris chart, the pancreas is situated at approximately 10, 20, 40, and 50 minutes, close to the collarette in both irides (see also Figure 6.7). It has eight reflex sites, four in each iris. The position in the left eye at 20 minutes is the *pancreas tail*, and this is the most important site to observe to check for a predisposition to Type 2 diabetes (this is where the insulin-producing beta cells in the Islets of Langerhans are found in greater proportions). A

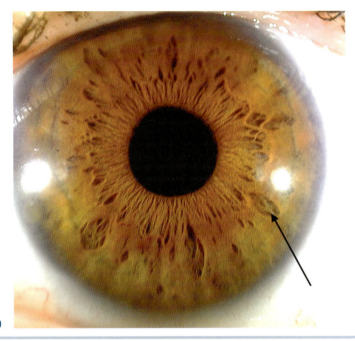

FIGURE 6.20

Leaf lacuna on the pancreas reflex at 20 minutes, left iris: possible family history of Type 2 diabetes.

lacuna here frequently shows a family history of diabetes (Figure 6.20).

The body and the head of the pancreas (left 40 minutes, right 20 minutes and 40 minutes) are more concerned with the provision of digestive juices and enzymes. The sites in the upper portion of the irides (left and right 10 minutes and 50 minutes) are considered to be secondary sites, and do not appear on some charts. However, it has been suggested that these reflect the posterior portion of the organ.

An additional marking for these sites is sometimes found in the "squaring" of the collarette, which also points to blood sugar issues (Figure 6.21). Additionally, bright orange pigments in the iris in any position are amplifying signs. (See "Pigmentation Signs," in Chapter 7.) Some researchers have suggested that a certain formation of lacuna, known as a "leaf lacuna," appearing anywhere in the region between 20 and 40 minutes in the humoral zone (just outside the collarette) may be interpreted as having pancreatic—and especially blood sugar—significance (Figure 6.22).

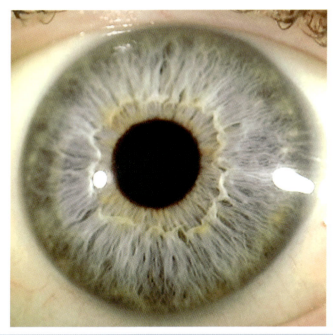

FIGURE 6.21

Square-shaped collarette—predisposing to blood sugar issues.

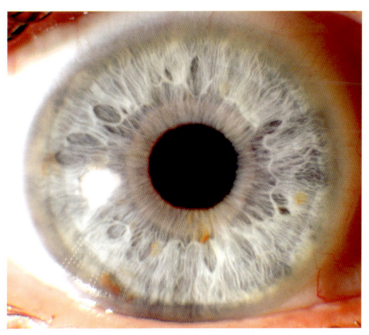

FIGURE 6.22

Lacunae on pancreatic positions and orange pigment distribution in a polyglandular iris.

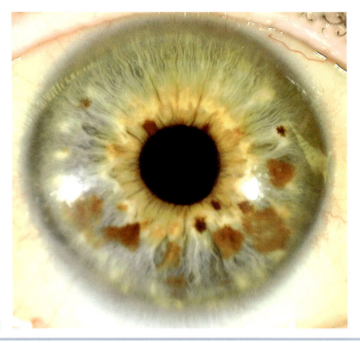

FIGURE 6.23

Distribution of topolabile brown pigment: implications towards liver congestion.

Emotional responses

A person's relationship toward anger, resentment, and frustration may also be revealed in these locations. The liver is the seat of many emotions, and imbalances in its function will often be tied in with failure to process these emotions effectively. Sometimes work on the liver will result in a welling up of such feelings, but this is a transitory reaction. The ability to mobilize emotions and release them is an important part of the way we assert ourselves in life. Persistent or stored anger (resentment) is linked to congestion of the liver, suggested by yellow and brown pigment (Figure 6.23), or by transversals, and should be regarded as a target for treatment, both physical and psychological. A denial of anger may be linked with insufficiency of the liver, seen in lacunae or rarefaction.

The heart

Situated in both irides at approximately 15 minutes and 45 minutes, close to the collarette, the heart is seen in several reflex areas. The position of the heart in the throat area (right iris 15 minutes and left iris 45 minutes) is important and reflects the embryological development of the organ, which takes place in what later becomes the throat (there is, particularly, a lifelong resonance between the heart and the thyroid gland—discussed at the end of this chapter). The major reflex site is in the left iris at 15 minutes, as the heart is mainly situated to the left of the body. But because it is close to the center of the body, we also see it reflected in the right iris at 45 minutes.

Lacunae in the heart zone are found fairly frequently, perhaps reflecting the fact that heart disease is still the biggest killer in our society. However, evidence of familial history of heart disease should not be regarded as a death sentence. It is a warning sign telling you to take care of your heart. A crypt or lacuna in the heart zone may be a sign that you need to embrace life joyfully and put your worries and anxieties to one side. Many heart attacks occur because people become isolated in their own worlds of worry and stress. To counteract this, it is necessary to relieve the pressure on the heart emotionally as well as physically.

You will note that the heart positions appear close to the border of the collarette, in the humoral zone, in the ring containing the other hormonal organs. This is highly significant. The heart actually secretes several key hormones that are especially involved on the management of stress through counteracting or opposing stress-related hormones such as cortisol, renin, and aldosterone, and having functions such as the relaxing and dilation of blood vessels, lowering blood pressure, and opening up access to the creative centers in the brain, particularly the hippocampus. (See Figure 6.24.) (You can find a thorough discussion of the heart-secreted hormones in the late Stephen Harrod Buhner's wonderful book, *The Secret Teachings of Plants*.[2])

The kidneys

Situated in the right iris at 28 to 31 minutes, and in the left iris at 29 to 32 minutes, the position of the kidneys on the chart may seem strange, being next to the leg in the lower portion of the iris. In the body, the kidneys are much higher up, in the mid-back area. However, their chart position reflects their embryological development.

The kidneys are very important to assess due to their role in filtering the blood and removing wastes. Alongside kidney function,

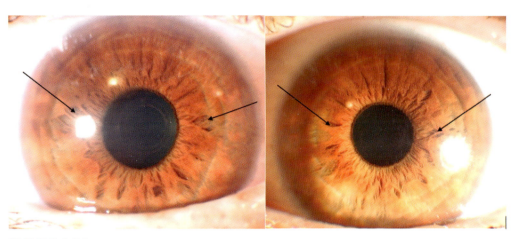

FIGURE 6.24

Lacunae/crypts in all four heart reflex positions: patient presented with atrial fibrillation.

we also need to assess the skin. If there is a scurf rim, the kidneys are probably doing extra work, and if they show signs of strain, then this needs to be addressed.

With a nod to Chinese medicine theory once more, it should be noted that lacunae or rarefaction in the kidney zones also can show a tendency to depletion and adrenal exhaustion, leading to chronic fatigue syndrome. Note the position of the adrenal glands at the apex of the kidney sector at 6 o'clock/30 minutes, close to the collarette in the humoral zone. (See Figure 6.25.)

Note also that the reflex area to the leg runs through the kidney zone at 30 minutes. If you see a sign along that line, you need to determine which part of the body is involved. A crypt at 30 minutes halfway out to the iris edge can alert you to either a kidney problem or a knee problem, so it will be important to cover both possibilities in your questioning.

The lungs and respiratory system

The reflex areas in the lateral outer ("temporal") sectors of the irides are given over largely to the lungs—although note the reflex sites for the breasts within the same field. Lacunae or rarefaction in this sector can indicate low resistance in the lungs and suggest the possibility of respiratory pathologies such as asthma and chronic obstructive pulmonary disease (COPD). (See Figure 6.26.)

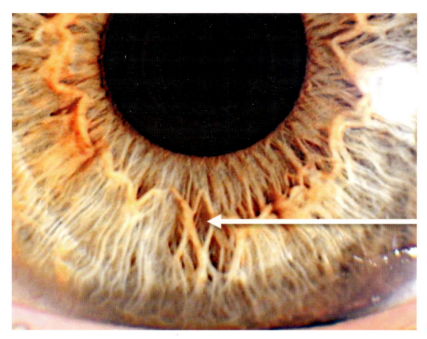

FIGURE 6.25

Crypts at adrenal and kidney locations.

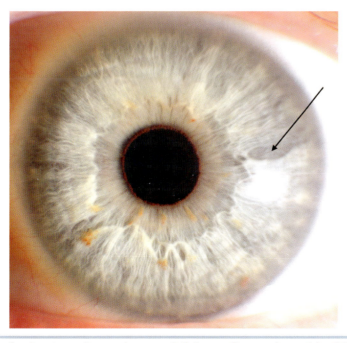

FIGURE 6.26

Rarefaction/open lacuna in upper left lung reflex: patient with a history of asthma.

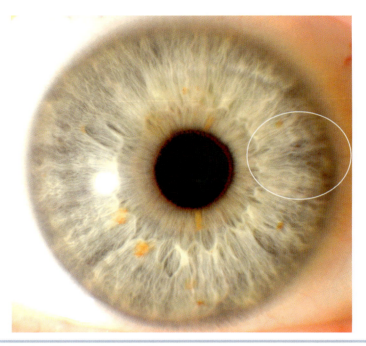

FIGURE 6.27

Rarefaction and irritation fibers in thyroid reflex zone:
family history of autoimmune thyroiditis.

In the inner lateral sectors (the "nasal" sectors) are found the reflex sites to the nose and the throat area, including the tonsils, the larynx, and the pharynx. Markings in these areas should be assessed for correlations involving a history of ear, nose, and throat (ENT) problems, but note also the reflex sites for the ears, on the opposite side of the iris disc at 7 minutes left and 53 minutes right.

The thyroid

You may already have noticed that the thyroid was not mentioned when discussing the humoral zone positions of the other hormonal organs. This is because almost every iris reflex chart places the thyroid outside the normal circuit, as it appears in the hormonal zone of the concentric chart, at approximately 45 minutes left and 15 minutes right and extending out almost to the iris margin.

It is not clear exactly why this is, in terms of the development of the chart; however, the position is validated again and again in practice, where signs in this sector are successfully matched to individual or family medical history. One possible answer has to do with the previous observation that heart and thyroid arise embryonically from the same bundle of tissue, before becoming separated as the anatomy develops. Maybe it is this separation, while retaining a strong sympathy or energetic connection, which is reflected in this rather off-key placing of the thyroid.

It is certainly true, however, that heart and thyroid maintain that close historic relationship throughout life: if you suffer with hypothyroidism (underactive thyroid), you will likely experience a slow heart rate (bradycardia); individuals with hyperthyroidism (overactive thyroid) will experience tachycardia, or a racing heartbeat. (See Figure 6.27.)

NOTES

1. Angerer, J. (1987). *Textbook of Eye Diagnosis.* Sydney: Institute of Research into Iris Studies.
2. Buhner, S. (2004). *The Secret Teachings of Plants in the Direct Perception of Nature.* Rochester, NY: Bear & Company.

7

The iris and its signs

The true individuality of the iris is discovered in the additional incidence of structural and pigmentation markings that make up the unique iris pattern.

Those markings and what they might mean is explored in this chapter. These signs are not to be interpreted strictly as indications of disease. Signs in the iris, like the overall constitutional indicators, are still to be considered as genetically inherited markers for certain tendencies or predispositions.

It has been calculated that there may be up to 200 differentiating signs in any iris, and with this amount of potential information at our disposal, we are going to need to know how to decide whether a sign is important or not.

This also brings forward another common problem that can afflict the unsuspecting beginner. There is a reason why, in presenting this material, I am keen to give a thorough grounding in the constitutional analysis before going into the labyrinthine territory of topographical markings.

The way I usually caution in class is to liken the focus on iris signs alone as looking for the trees at the expense of seeing the wood. The trees (iris signs) always exist in the context of the wood (the gestalt sum of the three levels of constitution). Starting with constitution enables us to construct a context in which signs, and potential problems, may be seen; we will often find that this context will assist us to identify the signs we really need to prioritize.

For example, say we have a hematogenic constitution with a lipemic diathesis, with its typical concerns around blood composition and cardiovascular risk factors. We then note a lacuna at 15 minutes in the left iris, the major heart zone. At that point, because of the hematogenic lipemic *context*, the weakness marking in the heart gains additional significance.

If we are unable to prioritize between the large number of iris signs potentially available, then we will find ourselves swamped with a bewildering array of pathological possibilities, which will not only confound our own ability to reach a coherent interpretation or reading but is highly likely to scare the patient—if not actually to make them ill! This is called "overdiagnosis" and has been the downfall of many an iridologist before now—in one instance on national television, when a program participant, having had her irides analyzed, was so alarmed by what she heard that she immediately checked herself into hospital for tests—which, of course, all came out normal. The subsequent verdict of the program regarding the practice of iridology was, understandably, somewhat unfavorable.

To be very clear, our diagnostic pronouncements are to be given in the contexts both of the full iris display, with its expression of the unique logic of every individual constitutional pattern, and of the presenting symptoms that the patient brings to the consultation and is asking for help with. Anything else risks being little more than conjecture, and while occasionally this may be accurate, we must still be extremely careful not to enact the "nocebo effect" (see Chapter 1).

The following three rules were taught to me in the early days, and I have always found them valuable. A sign should be regarded as potentially important if:

> ‣ it stands out and is immediately noticeable against the overall context of the iris display;
> ‣ it is amplified by other signs in the field, or by elements of the overall constitution;
> ‣ contrasting signs, or signs with opposite effects, are seen in the same iris zone or location—for example, light signs and dark signs together, or a lacuna sign and a pigment sign overlapping one another.

These rules are not exhaustive, but they serve as a useful immediate guide to triaging the large amount of information we are often faced with when first looking into any set of irides.

Signs are also not necessarily anchored to their topographical positions on the iris chart. There are two topographical orientations: *topostabile* signs are significant according to their position on the chart, while *topolabile* signs are significant for their general appearance and can occur anywhere on the chart, no matter what their meaning. This means that a brown pigment patch, for example, may point up issues with liver detoxification, even if it is found to be nowhere near the liver reflex. As a very general rule, structural signs are interpreted in a topostabile sense, and pigment signs—especially the pigment "freckles" found in many irides—are to be regarded as topolabile.

CATEGORIES OF IRIS SIGNS

For convenience, we group potential iris signs into three categories:

1. *Structural signs,* including lacunae and crypts, signs affecting the border of the collarette, and furrows
2. *Pigmentations signs,* involving secondary pigmentation not related to the basic eye color
3. Other signs, which is a catch-all to pick up on—for example, *ring signs, pupillary signs, scleral signs*

Structural signs: lacunae, crypts, and rarefactions

There are several types of lacunae, identified by size and shape. It is not my intention here to list and describe each one but, rather, to present the general conditions indicated and the therapeutic responses that they elicit. Generally, any disruption of iris texture potentially indicates an area where there is a need to restore, nourish, strengthen, stimulate, improve blood flow, enhance lymphatic drainage, and boost the flow of energy.

Closed lacuna

Most lacunae fall into this category (see Figure 7.1). These are completely encircled with a fibrous border, so that it looks like a hole in the texture. A closed lacuna may be regarded as a sign that one of your ancestors had a problem with the organ in that sector of the iris. A common example is a closed lacuna in the heart zone, which may show that a close forebear had heart disease or had suffered a heart attack. This does not mean you will have a heart attack, but you should be aware of a certain inherent susceptibility in the organ and avoid behavior that could exacerbate this.

Another common example is a "leaf lacuna" (a lesion that bears the shape of a leaf and may even have fibers within it that look like veins) at 20 minutes in the left iris. This is a well-known sign that suggests a family history of Type 2 diabetes. Again, you do not have to get the diabetes yourself, but we could also ask about predisposing factors, such as cravings for sweet things or bouts of low blood sugar. (A leaf lacuna on the adrenal signifies that stress may be involved in blood sugar problems: see Figure 7.2.)

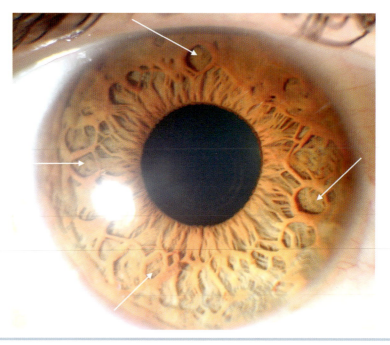

FIGURE 7.1

There are many closed lacunae in this iris: note the fibrous borders that completely encircle the arrowed lesions.

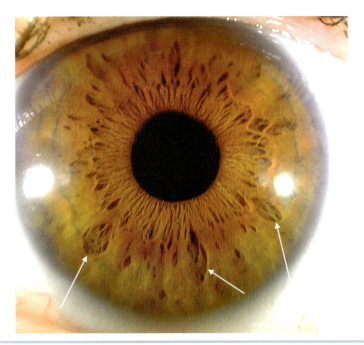

FIGURE 7.2

Leaf lacunae occur in this iris in pancreas positions (right and left) and at the adrenal reflex area (center).

Closed lacunae are therefore regarded as "genetic footprints": they do not have to be activated into pathology, but they may be if put under pressure.

Open lacuna

A hole in the texture that does not have a complete border and that has a section on the same level as the surrounding iris tissue is an *open lacuna* (Figure 7.3). While it indicates a potentially more serious situation—it points to a condition that may not yet have occurred or that is in process—you can still have plenty of influence over its development. For example, if you tend to have a recurrent chest complaint, you may find that you have an open lacuna (or rarefaction) in your lung zone.

The sign depicts a condition that needs to be healed. If you choose foods that strengthen the lungs and the immune system— such as garlic, onion, berries (for vitamin C and antioxidants), echinacea, wild cherry bark, elecampane, marshmallow, and

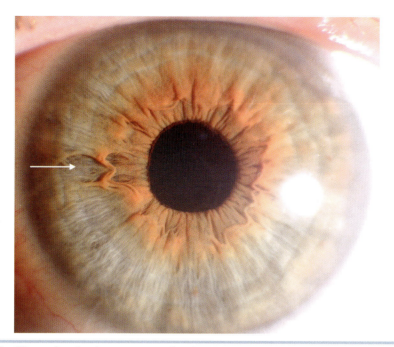

FIGURE 7.3

Open lacuna: the fibrous border does not completely encircle the lesion, leaving one side of it "open" to the surrounding iris tissue.

licorice—you will improve the organ's defenses and possibly avoid passing on problems to the next generation.

Remember, using antibiotics or other substances to suppress such a condition may store up trouble for later.

Depth of lacuna

Another important aspect of both open and closed lacunae is the depth of the hole. As we saw, the iris is composed of about four layers of fibers. Some lesions affect only the surface layer, with plenty of fibers visible within them; others penetrate to the deepest level, appearing darker or black. The deeper the penetration into the stroma, the more potentially "serious" the reading.

Lacunae may assume a variety of different shapes, and there are slightly different interpretations for each variation. However, the principles listed above give a good general understanding of how to interpret them.

Crypts and defects

A common example of a lacuna that penetrates to the deepest level of the iris is the crypt, which is small and often diamond-shaped. In Figure 7.4, the arrow points to a very deep "rhomboid" crypt. Many other lacuna structures can be seen in this iris, but they are quite shallow in comparison. Crypts are often found around the intestinal zone and are signs of the potential for degenerative conditions within the intestines, often involving parasite activity; wherever they are found, there will be risk for degenerative processes to set up over the course of life *if we do nothing to offset them.* See if you can spot more crypts in Figure 7.5.

A smaller version of the crypt is the "defect of substance" marking. This is regarded as a sign for chronic degenerative conditions. These markings are small, black pinprick holes that puncture to the deepest level. The smaller the hole, the more serious its significance may be. (See Figure 7.6.)

Crypts and defect markings may often be spotted inside larger lacunae. An example of this is the honeycomb lacuna, where a

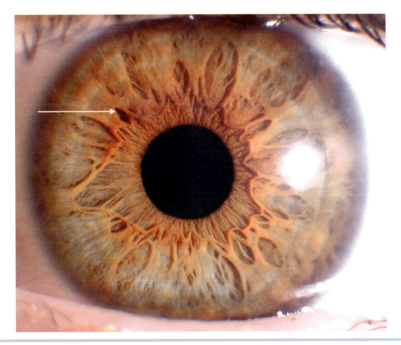

FIGURE 7.4

Very deep "rhomboid" (diamond-shaped) crypt.

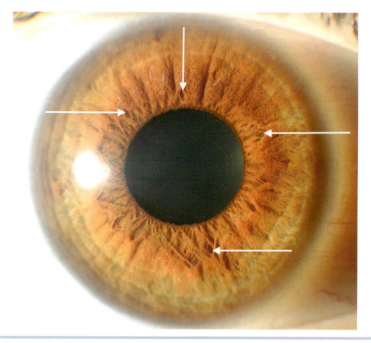

FIGURE 7.5

Crypts at the collarette border.

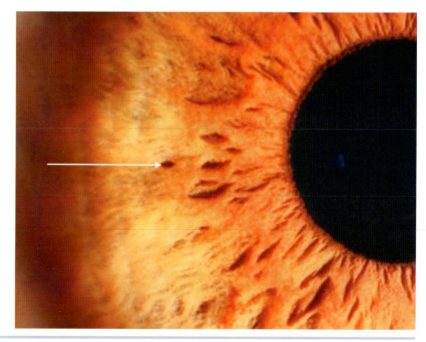

FIGURE 7.6

Defect of substance: a pinprick hole in the iris texture.

bordered lesion contains a network of smaller holes. These are often seen in the digestive zone and are considered signs for a terrain that invites parasitic infestation (Figure 7.7). Check for pain or feelings of bloating in the lower left abdominal region, which might flag up a parasite problem. If symptoms are found, research and carry out a herbal or naturopathic parasite cleanse (herbs might include wormwood, clove, and black walnut hulls). See also the bowel cleanse in Chapter 10.

Rarefactions

Rarefactions are variations in fiber density, but they have no fibrous border that defines their precise location. The fiber structure appears looser and darker, with a lower density and darker shading, implying reduced resistance and lowered vitality. Rarefactions often indicate that the vitality of an affected organ is low, giving rise to either functional or energetic deficit. (See Figure 7.8.)

For example, rarefaction in the lung zones is a well-known predisposing sign for asthma; rarefaction in a kidney zone may comment on the filtering capacity of the kidney but, equally, is

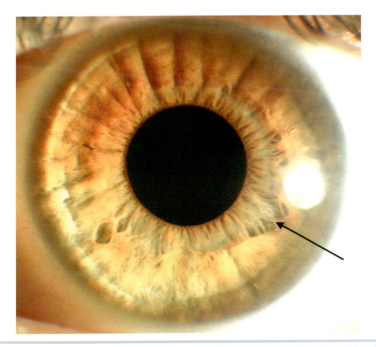

FIGURE 7.7

Honeycomb in the sigmoid colon reflex zone:

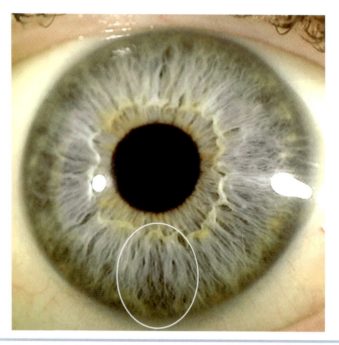

FIGURE 7.8

Fiber separation—"rarefaction"—in the kidney zone.

very often associated with fatigue and energy deficit; rarefaction in the thyroid zone can indicate hypothyroidism.

Learning from lacunae

On the one hand, lacunae are warning signs indicating reduced connective tissue integrity, leading potentially to poor nourishment, poor drainage, low immunity, and lowered local vitality and resistance, as well as to toxicity; parasite infestation, inherent organ weakness, ancestral disease patterns, organ insufficiency, and retention and accumulation.

They may, on the other hand, present opportunities for healing and for dispersing accumulated stress. They also point to receptivity, emotional honesty, creativity, and acceptance. Emotionally, they may also indicate vulnerability, confusion, a tendency to hand over their power to others too easily, and a lack of appropriate boundaries.

These structural signs will not change during life. They may occasionally look different due to fluctuations in pupil size, but they remain the same size and depth, and in the same positions, as when they crystallized in the eyes soon after birth. They can also serve as a map of certain lessons that perhaps need to be learned through life.

Signs affecting the border of the collarette

The border of the collarette (BC) is an important diagnostic tool that can deliver a wealth of information about the digestive tract and the autonomic nervous system—and the links between the two. Deviations in the appearance of the BC can have implications for the section of the digestive tract involved, but also for organs in the immediately adjacent zone outside the border.

Prominent, white, and hyperactive BC

This indicates hypersensitive intestinal mucosa and inflammatory reactions affecting the bowels, including food sensitivities and allergies, IBS symptoms, and even inflammatory bowel disease (IBD), which is an autoimmune condition. (See Figure 7.9.)

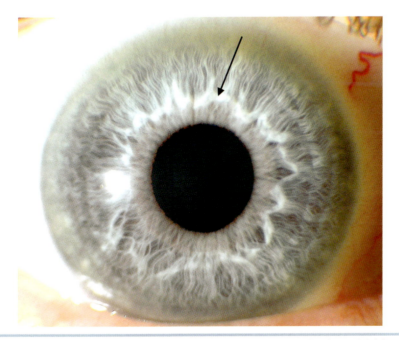

FIGURE 7.9

Bright white collarette border: IBS, food sensitivities, and allergies.

Exacerbating factors may be nervous tension, reduced digestive efficiency due to weakening of the liver, gallbladder, and pancreas, or disturbed gastrointestinal immunity. Use herbs such as chamomile, vervain, and skullcap to relax and soothe; deep breathing and hatha yoga (e.g., shoulder stand); visualization and relaxation.

Thin or invisible BC

A thin or invisible border of the collarette may indicate poor absorption and possible enzyme deficiency. Low visibility in the small intestine zone suggests problems with absorption of nutrients (Figure 7.10). You need to stimulate digestion and the production of digestive enzymes to improve the absorption and distribution of nutrients, and guard against sluggishness. Use bitters, spices, and pungent foods such as garlic, ginger, and cayenne in your food.

Expanded BC

An expanded collarette is discussed in "The Digestive-Regulatory Iris" section in Chapter 4, and it is shown in Figure 7.11. Note that an average placement for the collarette border is around a third the distance between the inner pupil border and the outer iris edge. Local protuberances containing deep lacunae within the collarette similarly warn of potential problems with gastrointestinal immunity—dysbiosis and parasites. Bowel cleanses should be used regularly.

Distensions of the border of the collarette also impact on the immediately adjacent area, where pressure arising within the digestive tract may adversely affect the organ in question. An example of this is so-called Römheld syndrome, which is where cardiac symptoms (e.g., chest pain, palpitations) may be experienced as a result of digestive disharmony. The iris pattern—known as cardio–abdominal syndrome—will show a distension of the collarette at 15 minutes left, and usually there will also be a marking in the heart zone just outside the collarette border. (See Figure 7.12.)

Contracted BC

A contracted collarette indicates spasmodic conditions affecting the digestive tract, along with low digestive capacity (Figure 7.13). The need here is to release and relax. Use tinctures or teas containing

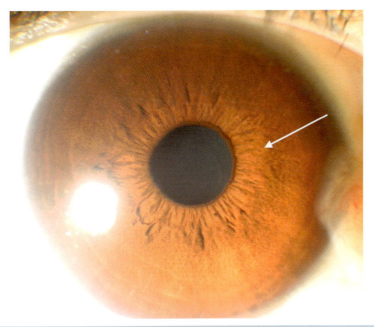

FIGURE 7.10

Low visibility of the collarette border around most of its circumference, especially in the small intestine zone.

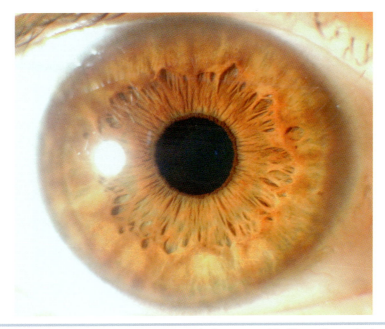

FIGURE 7.11

Gastric type: collarette border expanded to around half way from the inner pupil border to the edge of the iris.

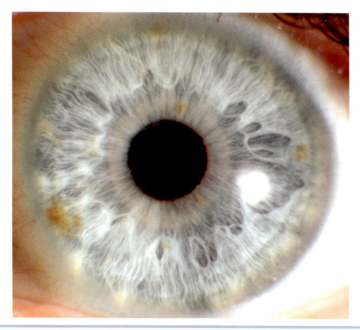

FIGURE 7.12

Cardio-abdominal syndrome: extreme collarette distension at 16–20 minutes (descending colon reflex), with crypts in the heart and aorta zones: possible Römheld syndrome.

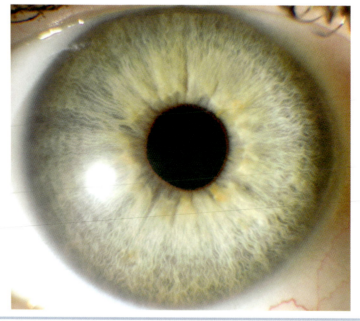

FIGURE 7.13

Contracted collarette border: spasmodic conditions affecting digestion, low enzyme provision and low digestive capacity.

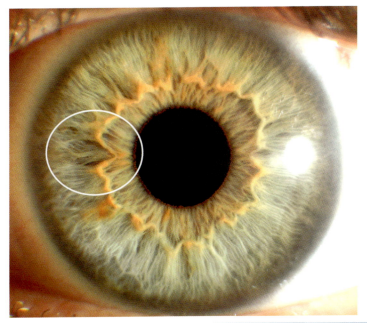

FIGURE 7.14

Local indentation of the collarette border at 45 minutes, with open lacuna in the adjacent sector.

skullcap, passionflower, wild yam, or black cohosh, and gentle laxatives such as linseed, psyllium, and slippery elm, taken as powders mixed with water or juice. Also try carminative herbs, such as fennel seed and angelica root, to increase digestive power, and apply "mealtime hygiene" principles (see "Mixed Biliary" discussion, Chapter 3). Again, localized contractions may also indicate spasmodic conditions affecting the organ in the adjacent sector of the ciliary zone. In Figure 7.14, note the open lacuna/honeycomb in the heart/throat/thyroid sector, and check for problems in those organs.

Individual fiber signs

Irritation fiber

A prominent, bright, or white fiber running from the collarette to the iris edge signifies irritation and reactivity in the organ represented in that portion of the iris. (It should be borne in mind that these signs are very small and are generally only visible in lighter iris types).

Irritation fiber in the left eye at 14–15 minutes or the right at 44–45 minutes reveals a potential for stress-related (neurogenic) heart disease. In a mixed iris an irritation fiber in the right iris at around 40 minutes can show gallbladder problems. In Figure 7.15, showing an irritation fiber, there is also a lipemic diathesis (cholesterol ring), so stress affecting the heart must be considered.

Transversal fibers

A transversal fiber runs across the grain of the iris instead of in a radial direction out toward the edge. These were once thought to indicate trauma or accidental damage; however, this is difficult to prove as we would need to demonstrate that they were not there before the trauma took place. They are associated with acute or chronic inflammation and potential tissue changes.

Transversals may come in several patterns, some of which are

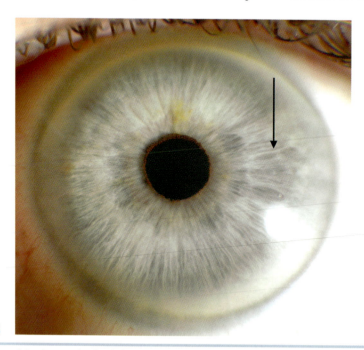

FIGURE 7.15

Irritation fiber at 14 minutes in the left iris, and a lipemic diathesis (cholesterol ring).

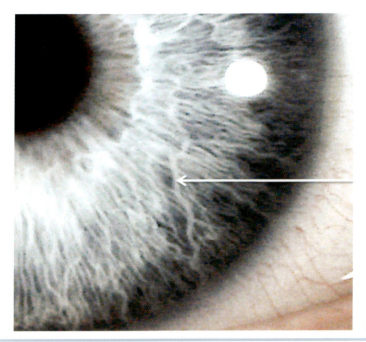

FIGURE 7.16

Spleen-heart transversal fiber: possible family history of heart problems.

regarded as relatively serious. An example of this is the so-called "spleen–heart" transversal, seen in the left iris, which is a sign for a possible risk or family history of heart attack (Figure 7.16).

Where you see a transversal fiber, support is needed for the local organ, but also for the whole system, to reduce inflammation and promote healing.

Vascularized fibers

Sometimes a blood vessel within the iris may engorge with blood, and its outer sheath can split away, revealing a pink thread. Vascularization may be a sign of physical trauma affecting the organ indicated, or it might be a sign of a buried emotional trauma. I have seen these signs several times in the children of alcoholics—noting their appearance in the liver and spleen region, in particular. Ask about any obvious symptoms, and treat the cause. (See Figure 7.17.)

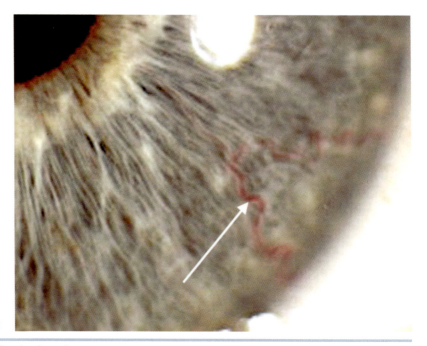

FIGURE 7.17

Vascularized fiber in the spleen zone.

Herbal choices

For trauma and wound healing: St John's Wort, comfrey (external use only), marigold, arnica (external use only, except homeopathically), aloe vera.

For cooling and soothing nerves: Skullcap, vervain, passionflower.

Furrow types

Contraction and radial furrows are defining components of the self-protective iris, where we see these signs in abundance. However, they can also be seen as individual signs in any iris type.

Contraction furrows

Also known as *concentric* or *circular* furrows, these signs look like ripples in the surface of the iris and can be partial or plentiful, extending around the iris disc in a concentric pattern. Sometimes also called "nerve rings," they are signs of nervous tension and a tendency to internalize stress and to use nutritional energy up quickly. Eat carefully and regularly, and do not become exhausted.

Look for breaks in the rings: these are the points where stress may be causing problems to the organ in question. However, in a dense iris with few other structural signs, they may be the only opportunities for the release of stress and are possibly similar in meaning to lacunae or rarefactions in a less dense iris. In case of a break like the one shown in Figure 7.18, check for signs of stress affecting kidney or adrenal function, including fatigue.

Look for (sometimes unacknowledged) neuromuscular tension held deep within the body tissues, and a tendency to internalize stress.

Radial furrows

Radial furrows come in two forms: major radials, which start at the pupil edge and cut through the collarette as they point

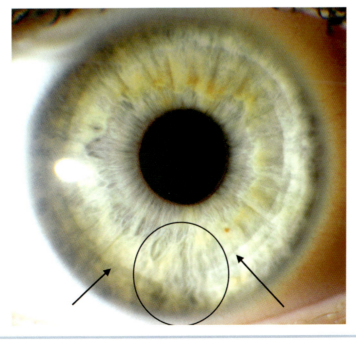

FIGURE 7.18

Break in contraction furrows in the kidney zone.

toward the outer iris edge; and minor radials, which start at the collarette (Figure 7.19). Major radials imply a weakening of the ANS. Radials are both a sign of potential for toxic leakage from a congested bowel and a sign of nerve weakness, particularly affecting the gastrointestinal tract, but also the radial zone in which they are seen.

In a digestive context they are also known as "spasm furrows" and may be associated with bouts of actual abdominal pain or spasm. Spastic constipation may be a tendency; if confirmed, use relaxants and antispasmodics, rather than stimulating laxatives. Magnesium may be given.

Also in a digestive context, major radials in particular can indicate leaky or permeable gut syndrome. Here the furrows seem to represent deep channels through which toxic material can gain access to the surrounding circulatory channels and thus affect the whole body. In this context it would be well to remember that stress and tension are directly contributory to leaky gut syndrome.

Radial furrows in the upper zone (brain reflex area) can indicate headache, neck pain, insomnia, and a tendency to "overthink" (Figure 7.20).

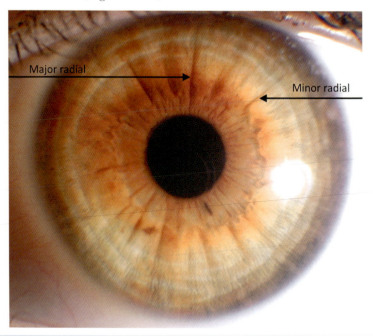

FIGURE 7.19

Major and minor radials.

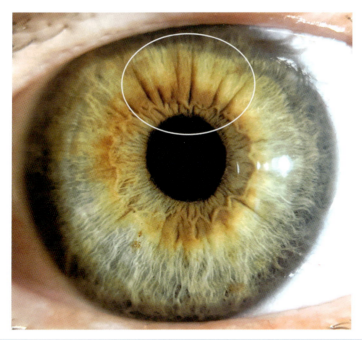

FIGURE 7.20

Radial furrows in the upper zone.

Treatment for contraction and radial furrows

Massage and relaxing body work is highly effective for contraction furrows, as is acupuncture and other forms of energetic balancing and adjustment. As these furrows also suggest increased utilization of nutrients, checking for and treating digestive weaknesses is important. For radial furrows, consider a bowel cleansing program in order to ensure that bowel toxins, which should be released through defecation, do not gain access to the interior. (See Chapter 10.)

PIGMENTATION SIGNS

Pigment signs are regarded as the opposite of lacunae in terms of meaning: whereas lacunae signify insufficiency, pigment signifies excess, concentration, and crystallization.

Learning from pigmentation

Pigmentation of the whole iris determines constitutional type, but spots or flecks of pigment or sections of different color also can occur in the iris. These pigments are usually deposits in the anterior border layer, the transparent film that encases the iris. Pigments can indicate an accumulation of potentially toxic pollutants or metabolic wastes; a sluggishness or blockage of energy in affected organs or systems; a tendency to excess and crystallization, such as gallstones or kidney stones; tissue changes (shown by darker colors); a reduced flow of digestive enzymes; and protection of organs from excess stimulation by heat or light.

Pigments can also indicate resistance, self-protection, repression of emotions, obsessive thoughts and fears, an analytical or intellectual nature, secrecy, passion, aggression, insight, organizational abilities, and a strongly visual approach to learning.

Treatment for pigmentation signs

Useful treatments are those that disperse accumulations and remove blockages, such as deep-tissue detoxification and therapies that move energy: polarity therapy, shiatsu, or acupuncture. Treatments that break up deposits, such as packs and poultices (see Chapter 10), can be applied to sites of cysts, polyps, tumors, calcification, pain, stiffness, and inflammation.

Since pigments also frequently denote reduced enzyme provision, especially from liver and pancreas, treatments should also include herbs and foods that support these organs: digestive stimulants such as gentian root, barberry bark, citrus peel and fennel seed, mild spices in food, and fresh-squeezed juices should be given. Use the pigment differentiation chart (Table 7.1) as a guide to which organs to support.

Classifying pigments

Other examples of this kind of pigment are the central and sectoral heterochromia. A *central heterochromia* is, literally translated, a "different color in the middle", and a *sectoral heterochromia* is a radial section of a different color. These appearances are

Table 7.1   Iris pigment differentiation chart

Color	Organ	Description and interpretation
Pale or straw yellow	Kidneys	Occurs as diffuse pigment throughout the iris. Can indicate bowel toxicity due to poor breakdown of animal proteins, and resultant stress on kidneys. Amplifies hyperacidic type.
Bright yellow	Liver	Spots or patches inside and outside the collarette, as central heterochromia and in plaques and flocculations. Intolerance to rich, fatty foods (dairy), difficulty with fat metabolism.
Orange-yellow/ ocher	Liver/ gallbladder	The more concentrated the color, the more the diathesis moves toward the gallbladder. Gallstones, biliary colic, cholecystitis.
Bright orange	Pancreas	Spots and patches throughout the iris, often with an uneven or grainy appearance, signs for blood sugar issues.
Salmon red	Stomach	Patches and spots usually found within the stomach zone, often very small. Disturbances of stomach enzymes and secretions. Possibility of ulceration or malignancy.
Brown/ red brown	Liver	Patches, spots, central heterochromia. Problems with the detoxifying functions of the liver–CYP enzymes (phase 1 liver detoxification). Liver congestion.
Dark brown	Liver/colon	As above, but extending also into the intestine, where detoxifying CYP enzymes are also found. Disturbances of liver function, constipation, autointoxication.
Black or "tar" pigments	Lymph/ immunity	Spots and freckles scattered throughout the iris— can also be seen in hematogenic types. Lymphatic stasis, immune suppression, depression and melancholy, overthinking.

topostabile: they usually affect the organs in that iris sector. For example, a central heterochromia highlights the digestive tract.

Yellow-orange central heterochromia (liver/gall bladder affectations) is shown in Figure 7.21. Note also the thickness and prominence of the BC (food sensitivities): check for maldigestion or symptoms when eating fatty foods, especially dairy produce.

Orange sectoral heterochromia in the throat/thyroid zone is shown in Figure 7.22. Note also the small grey rarefaction in the center of the zone: check for problems affecting this area of the body, including difficulties vocalizing or expressing feelings. Digestion may also be involved: digestive deficiency gives rise to excess phlegm production."

Changing colors?

Pigments are considered to be largely genetically determined and therefore not subject to change, contrary to what many would like to think. Pigments are part of individuals' uniqueness. Imagine

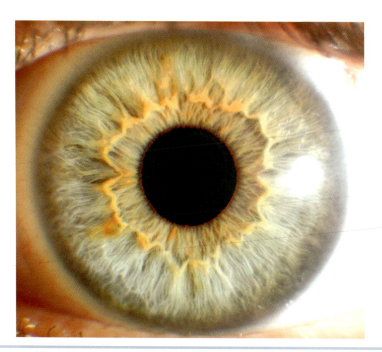

FIGURE 7.21

Yellow-orange central heterochromia (liver/gall bladder affectations).

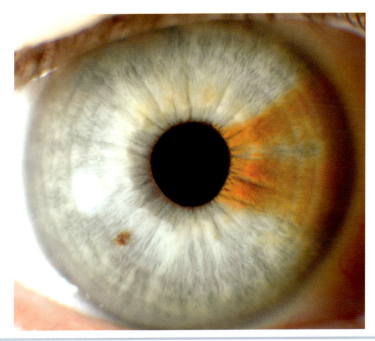

FIGURE 7.22

Orange sectoral heterochromia in the throat/thyroid zone.

if you could remove them by "detoxing": what would happen when you next relied on them for bio-identification purposes? You might not be able to access you bank account, or make it through passport control!

Psychologically, pigment shows considerable disposition toward mental activity and analysis. The darker the pigment, the greater the tendency to brooding and obsessiveness. Those with a scattering of very dark brown or black spots (called tar pigments) often need help with escaping from their thoughts. If you see tar pigments, such as those shown in Figure 7.23, check for appropriate immune activation, as well as for signs of internalized stress, melancholy, and brooding tendencies. This tendency may also be a cause of serious disturbance or suppression, particularly of immunity. Often people with these signs report hardly ever getting sick with "infections". This is not necessarily good news: it may simply be that immunity is suppressed and unable to mount a reaction. However, when people of this type are in balance, they are great thinkers, intellectuals, scientists, and analysts.

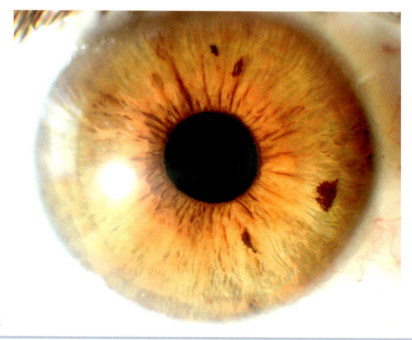

FIGURE 7.23

Tar pigments.

RING SIGNS

In this section we round up the chapter by mentioning a few of the additional signs and appearances that can lead us to important diagnostic information.

The scurf rim

In pale blue eyes a dark band at the outer edge of the iris—the scurf rim—can often be seen clearly without the aid of a magnifier. It is very common to the hyperacidic type and also to the rheumatic type. Literally, it is rarefaction of iris fiber structure, affecting the outer zone.

If you see a scurf rim, such as that shown in Figure 7.24, check for skin issues, like eczema or dry or itchy skin.

This sign indicates that the skin is underactive, is not discharging well, and may become overloaded and congested. This may manifest in the form of an outbreak—eczema, psoriasis, acne, or sensitivity, itchiness, and dryness.

The outer zone of the iris is the zone of elimination: darkness or rarefaction in this zone (see section above, "Structural Signs: Lacunae, Crypts, and Rarefactions") depict poor elimination, which results in a buildup and overloading of toxins and must be tackled via a suitable therapeutic program. Stimulating the skin will also relieve pressure on the kidneys, which may be struggling to cope with excessive elimination. Psychologically, there is a tendency to hold in emotions, especially irritation and anger, suppression of which may be a direct cause of skin outbreaks. This should be taken into consideration in the treatment.

The skin is our physical interface with the environment, and skin eruptions tend to imply some suppression of feelings concerning our interactions with the world and with others. We may not express this verbally or behaviorally, but our system may express

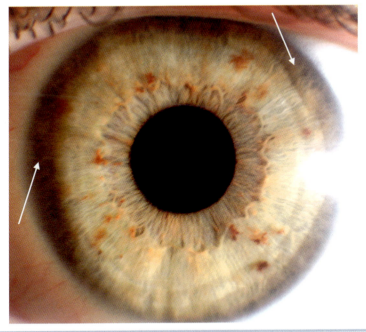

FIGURE 7.24

Dark outer zone: the *scurf rim.*

it in an outbreak of some kind, possibly on our skin. Examine feelings of anger or resentment and try to come to terms with them. Work on feeling safe. Skin problems also can imply a lack of trust in others and an inability to express negative feelings.

Treatment for the scurf rim

Use dry skin brushing or other forms of exfoliation, such as aduki bean scrubs. Also, hydrotherapy—the use of hot and cold water—stimulates the skin, as do saunas, steam baths, and Turkish baths; don't forget to use the cold plunge between bouts in the hot rooms. If you have cardiovascular problems, ask a health professional what course of action would be appropriate, as sudden extremes of temperature may cause shock and exacerbate existing pathologies.

Herbal choices

Mountain grape root and burdock are both blood-cleansing herbs that work on the liver and kidneys and have a special affinity with the skin. Red clover flowers, calendula flowers, rose petals, cleavers, and passionflower can all be combined into a very effective floral skin-clearing tea that is pleasant to take as well as effective for conditions such as eczema.

Elderflower, peppermint or spearmint, and yarrow and ginger are good to promote perspiration. These herbs are best taken as teas.

For dry and itchy skin use chickweed, calendula, and oat straw (or porridge oats) in a bath: place the herbs in a muslin bag and allow to infuse before entering the bath.

The anemia ring

This ring appears as a fuzzy or blurred edge to the iris, often in the upper sectors, but occasionally found all the way around the iris disk. It represents lack of definition at the boundary between the tissue of the iris and the sclera (the limbus).

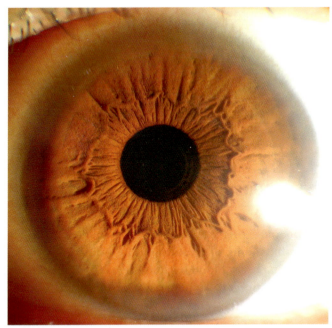

FIGURE 7.25.

A fuzzy, indistinct iris margin in the upper sector.

In the case of a blurred edge to the iris, such as shown in Figure 7.25, check for anemia and cognitive difficulties.

This ring indicates a possible failure of the blood to oxygenate or nourish the peripheral tissues. In the cerebral region, this can lead to problems with memory and mental function (brain fog). In an advanced state it can signify a more general anemic condition; however, in more generally applicable terms it maps very clearly to the Chinese medicine pathologic state known as *blood deficiency*. (See also "The Hematogenic Constitution," in Chapter 3.)

Treatment

Eat foods that nourish the blood, such as dark green vegetables, beetroot and beetroot greens, and spinach; red fruits (high in antioxidants for blood cleansing); sprouted alfalfa seeds; and spirulina, chlorella, and other chlorophyll-rich foods (chlorophyll is chemically similar to hemoglobin).

Herbal choices

Blood-nourishing and iron-rich herbs   nettle leaf, Dong Quai, European angelica, astragalus, yellow dock root, raspberry leaf, bilberry fruit.

To improve blood flow to the extremities   Ginger, cayenne, and ginkgo.

The venous ring

A vivid blue ring around the outer edge of the iris may flag up sluggishness and congestion of the venous circulation—that is, the vessels that carry blood back to the heart and lungs for gas exchange.

If you observe a blue ring around the iris, such as that in Figure 7.26, check for varicose veins and/or hemorrhoids.

This results in poor elimination of carbon dioxide and acid

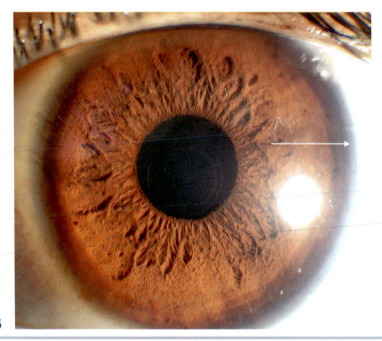

FIGURE 7.26

A blue tinge at the border of the iris (limbus) denotes the venous ring.

wastes, as the venous blood has problems returning to the heart and lungs to discharge the wastes and become reoxygenated. As a consequence, this can also suggest poor oxygenation of tissues.

This sign is seen most frequently in the hematogenic iris, where it amplifies constitutional concerns, but it is found in all iris types. The sign indicates a need to check for signs of stagnation or sluggishness affecting the liver or the bowel, as this "core congestion" may be responsible for back-pressure that is preventing the venous blood from returning efficiently to the cardiopulmonary system.

The most presenting common symptoms that you need to ask about where you see this ring are varicose veins and hemorrhoids.

Treatment for the venous ring

The circulation needs to be stimulated and blood moved more efficiently. Inverted yoga postures and the use of slant-boards or equipment that enables a reversal of the normal gravitational direction are effective.

Herbal choices

Garlic, ginger, and cayenne stimulate and cleanse the blood and circulation; red clover thins and cleanses the blood; hawthorn improves the elasticity of vessels; and horse chestnut is effective for varicose veins, including hemorrhoids, which often accompany this condition. These herbs are usually taken as tinctures.

Pupil size and shape

Sympathetic and parasympathetic nerve impulses control pupil size, and shape deviations inform about the nervous system (see Chapter 2).

A continuously enlarged pupil can indicate a person with a tendency to adrenal hyperactivity, who is always on the go and is quite sociable but finds it difficult to shut down. Extreme expansion of the pupils portends adrenal exhaustion and chronic

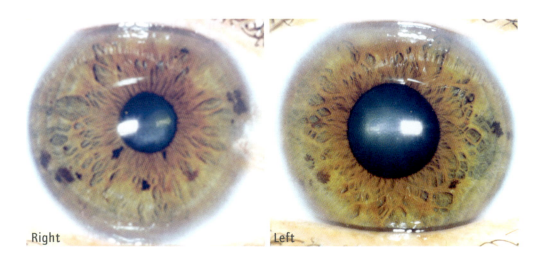

Right   Left

FIGURE 7.27

Pupils of unequal size—*anisocoria*.

fatigue. A permanently contracted pupil may indicate that a person is introverted, generally sluggish, has slow reactions, and lacks enthusiasm. When the sympathetic nervous system is weak, the parasympathetic is dominant, and vice versa. Treatment should work to moderate the dominant system and strengthen the weaker system.

Occasionally a person may have pupils of differing sizes (anisocoria) (Figure 7.27). This can indicate a family history of syphilis, diphtheria, or meningitis: check for any signs of compromise to the nervous and immune systems. It can also indicate Horner syndrome: a condition in which an injury to the nerves causes one pupil to become permanently smaller than the other. In this case the discrepancy is acquired, not natal.

Generally, deviations in any of the circular structures of the iris will potentially reveal information about the nervous system. The pupil may have areas of flatness around its circumference, and the adjacent iris sector may show evidence of problems in the organ represented in that sector, so consult the iris chart for more information. If a problem exists, consider the possibility that nerve supply may be involved, perhaps originating in a misalignment of the spine placing pressure on nerve pathways.

THE SPINAL MAP

You can use the pupil margin as a map of the spine. Divide each pupil in half by drawing a line from top to bottom. Each half represents the spinal column, with the cervical spine at the top, the thoracic in the midsection, and the lumbar and sacral vertebrae in the lower segment, in each half. A spinal misalignment may be assumed from any section that is flattened (see above): simply estimate which area of the spine is involved. If the same flatness is in both pupils, the indication is reinforced (Figures 7.28 and 7.29).

In addition, spinal misalignments can also be involved in patterns of disharmony affecting the internal organs. My friend and colleague, the late Peter Bradbury of the Guild of Naturopathic Iridologists, self-published a highly useful guide to pupil dynamics, taking in both spinal and visceral interpretations.[1]

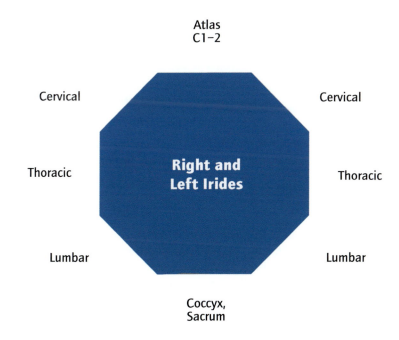

FIGURE 7.28

Simplified diagram of spinal sections mapping to patterns of pupillary flattening.

Table 7.2   Psychological interpretations

Signs	Interpretation
Digestive signs (concentric zones 1 and 2)	Self-nourishment and the willingness (or not) to give and receive unconditional love; a yearning for a love that can never be satisfied due to a lack of belief that one deserves it or is capable of receiving it; eating disorders; an energetic connection to the earth.
Kidney and pelvic signs (bottom or ventral sector)	Self-determination and individuation; your creative potential; self-confidence; the role of fear in your upbringing, whether of punishment or of not being well supported or appreciated; conditional love—striving to achieve in order to prove worthiness.
Liver, gallbladder, pancreas, and spleen signs (20 minutes and 40 minutes)	Anger, resentment, or frustration, and expressing these emotions; depression; capitulation to the demands of others (lacunae or rarefaction); boastful self-confidence that masks low self-esteem (pigment); perfectionism; assertiveness.
Lung signs (temporal sectors)	The ability (or not) to develop intimate relationships; an ability to share, expand toward others, and receive their expansion toward you; willingness to nourish yourself emotionally and physically (oxygen is a primary nutrient).
Heart and throat signs (nasal sectors, heart reflexes: left, 15 minutes and right, 45 minutes)	Honest expression; grief and yearning for union, both universal and human; isolation and separation; the ability or not to open up to life with joy and abandon.
Head area signs (top or frontal sector)	Depression, melancholy, moodiness (a lacuna at the pineal gland reflex can indicate Seasonal Affective Disorder[SAD syndrome]); preoccupation and obsession (pigments and radial furrows); spiritual dimension—a lacuna can signify spiritual opening or revelation, psychic abilities, or a strong religious or spiritual direction, often arrived at after emotional or psychological difficulty.

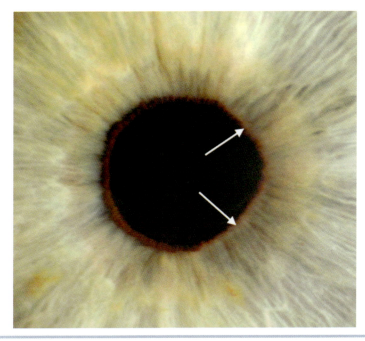

FIGURE 7.29

Examples of pupil flattening, probably in this case signifying problems with the upper thoracic and lumbar sections of the spine.

Psychological interpretations

Indications in the iris may also be significant emotionally or psychologically, rather than physically or physiologically.

Table 7.2 shows a brief overview of psychological interpretations for different types of signs in the iris and the issues they highlight. There is not space in this book to explore this application of iridology in detail, but a future volume will be devoted to this layer of iris interpretation.

NOTE

1. Bradbury, P. (1994). *Pupillotonia & Pupil Manifestations*. London: Guild of Naturopathic Iridologists.

8

Assessing your iris

By now you may have examined your eyes and discovered some signs, compared them with the iris chart, and perhaps started to think, "Help! I'm falling apart!" Bear in mind that a sign does not indicate a disease: most of the signs that you might see in your irides may never become physical problems. Signs should not be interpreted literally without reference to your symptoms, lifestyle, and medical history, and your family or ancestral medical history. To avoid overdiagnosis, you need to learn how to assess the importance of the signs observed, and how to place them in the context of your life.

An iridology assessment also can direct you to other tests and exploratory procedures that may shed light on your situation. In addition, because iridology concentrates on the causal factors in producing illness, it can help you to determine how to reverse the disease process and begin the journey back to health. Even in cases of known degenerative illness, iridology can suggest ways in which health may be safely improved. I've included some standard checklists that will help you to make sense of what you see and make a balanced assessment, as opposed to interpreting signs strictly according to "illnesses" that they supposedly indicate. The order of consideration is: symptoms, case history, iris display.

MAKING A HEALTH ASSESSMENT

Usually, we visit a doctor or health professional because we are experiencing symptoms and, having described these symptoms, the practitioner uses them to form an initial assessment of the problem. This is called *differential diagnosis*; it is the process of determining what the problem is most likely to be by reference to outward signs. The advantage of this approach is the recognition that a pain in, for example, the left arm will not necessarily indicate a problem with that arm: the pain may be due, for example, to angina, a serious and potentially life-threatening cardiovascular problem. Differential diagnosis is a medical skill that needs to be learned in an appropriate training context. However, symptoms also are likely to be the most common starting point in a self-evaluation, and they must be taken into account. Symptoms are the body's primary means of communicating its inner distress. Always listen and take note, and then try to find out what they mean.

Remember that the meaning of an iris sign may not always be entirely physical. Emotional or psychological concerns may also be at the root. Try to treat the whole picture, otherwise you could well overlook important causal factors, and your condition, even if it initially responds to therapy, may well recur.

Assessing your symptoms

Divide your body into separate anatomical systems, and study each one: skin, muscles, bones, nerves and brain, hormones, digestion, kidneys and urinary tract, respiratory tract, immune system, heart and circulation, and reproductive organs.

Write down each system as a separate heading, and then make a note of whatever you notice about each category, including positive factors as well as negative ones.

Creating a case history

After listing any symptoms, compile a case history. This can be created at any time, but set aside sufficient time for it, as it is important to create a thorough and comprehensive survey of lifestyle, medical history, and family patterns. Make notes in the categories listed below.

In your self-evaluation, list your symptoms and any important details about your habits, previous illnesses, family medical history, medications, etc., creating a thorough survey.

Main symptoms currently experienced

If you have multiple symptoms, it is best to come up with a shortlist of three or four main symptoms. You can note any other small symptoms in Table 8.1.

Medical history:

> Personal medical history from childhood, including vaccinations, hospitalizations, surgery, medication (including current), etc.

> Family medical history back to grandparents: what illnesses did they suffer; if they have died, how old were they and what did they die of?

> If you have children, their medical histories.

> Any previous experience of alternative or complementary medicine, including homeopathy, acupuncture, osteopathy, or herbalism.

> Any dietary supplements taken: herbs, homeopathic medicines, vitamins, minerals, etc.

Lifestyle:

> Your diet: draw up a chart detailing what you usually eat daily for breakfast, lunch, and dinner, and any snacks or drinks, etc. Pay particular attention to how often and how much you eat of potential problem-causing foods, such as

Table 8.1.   Anatomical system of the body

System	Organs/parts of body involved	Function	Your symptoms
Integumentary	Skin, hair, nails	Protection, regulation of heat, excretion	
Lymphatic	Lymph vessels and channels, spleen lymph nodes, lymphoid aggregations (e.g., tonsils, appendix), lymphatic fluid, lymphocytes	Recycling and cleansing of body fluids, immunity	
Musculo-skeletal	Muscles, tendons, ligaments, bones	Movement, protection, stabilization of posture, generation of heat	
Cardiovascular	Heart, arteries, veins, capillaries, blood—red and white corpuscles, spleen, lungs	Oxygenation and nourishment of tissues, maintenance of blood pressure	
Digestive	Mouth, teeth, esophagus, stomach, small and large intestines, bowel, liver, gallbladder, pancreas, digestive secretions	Assimilation of nutrients, production of energy	
Respiratory	Mouth, ears, nose, larynx, pharynx, trachea bronchi, lungs, heart	Oxygenation, excretion	

System	Organs/parts of body involved	Function	Your symptoms
Reproductive– Female	Uterus, fallopian tubes, ovaries, vagina, breasts	Procreation, sexuality	
Reproductive– Male	Penis, testes, prostate	Procreation, sexuality	
Hormonal (endocrine)	Pituitary, thyroid, parathyroid, pancreas, adrenals, gonads, other organs also having hormone receptors	Communication, regulation, metabolism	
Nervous	Brain, spinal column, nerves, eyes	Communication, sensation, movement, thought, and feeling	
Immune	Lymph, leucocytes, phagocytes, lymphoid aggregations (tonsils, adenoids), other organs having receptors: pervasive system	Protection and defense against pathogens, tumor surveillance, inflammatory capacity	
Urinary	Kidneys, ureters, bladder, urethra, penis	Excretion of waste products, temperature regulation	

dairy products, wheat, and yeast (the most common food allergens). Note any shortfall of fluid intake (especially water), and the amount of tea and coffee drunk. Also note down your consumption of animal proteins (list what kinds of meats are eaten, and if organically farmed).

▷ Past dietary patterns or habits.

▷ Other habits—e.g., smoking, alcohol intake, and use of recreational drugs.

▷ Your job and work history; list any work-related stresses that you experience, now or in the past.

▷ Personal relationships: current and previous stresses relating to family and friends, and past emotional trauma or bereavements.

▷ Your emotional and mental life: level of satisfaction in life, hobbies, or other pursuits. Do you balance your work, rest, and play?

▷ Any spiritual beliefs or experiences you have or have had.

Physical functions ("systems checks"):

▷ Digestion: appetite, indigestion or bloating, flatulence, acid reflux, frequency and consistency of bowel motions.

▷ Cardiovascular health: blood pressure, heart rate, cholesterol levels (if known) general circulation (e.g., cold hands or feet).

▷ Nervous system: sleep patterns, cognitive function (memory and concentration), symptoms affecting hearing or vision, any tingling or numbness, pins and needles, headaches or migraine.

▷ Immune system: frequency of contracting infections, length of time typically taken to recover, allergies, healing abilities.

▷ Respiratory system—shortness of breath, asthma, ear–nose–throat problems including sinuses.

▷ Skin—dry or moist, outbreaks or rashes, dandruff or scurf.

▷ Urinary system—recurrent urinary tract infections, water retention.

▷ Reproductive (female)—painful periods, PMS, ovarian cysts, fibroids, fertility, libido.

▷ Reproductive (male)—prostate (urine stream), premature ejaculation, impotence and erectile dysfunction, libido.

➢ Musculoskeletal—joint aches or pains, muscle aches, stiffness/inflammation, muscular strength, bone density.
➢ Hormonal—thyroid, blood sugar balance, vitality and energy (adrenals).

IRIS DISPLAY

Having made your inventory of symptoms and personal history, you are ready to assess your iris display. Start with the basic constitution associated with your irides: blue, brown-eyed, or mixed (Chapter 3). Then assess the structure of your irides (Chapter 4), and finally the overlay or diathesis (Chapter 5).

Then list the four or five signs that stand out to you, and their meanings, for example, lacunae or crypts, pigments, contraction furrows, a scurf rim, or bright white signs. You may find that certain patterns or themes begin to appear. Don't tackle more than four or five signs at first, and choose obvious ones. You also need to assess your energy, stamina, and any other, possibly underlying, influences that may be potential threats that put pressure on the organs or systems that are flagged up.

The squint test

This is a simple way of determining which iris signs are important. You need to squint as you look, blurring your vision. You will immediately lose the details and be left with the most obvious features. The following guidelines will help you choose those that need further exploration (see also Chapter 7):

1. A sign stands out (e.g., a large lacuna, a big black pigment, or an orange central heterochromia against a blue/gray background). If something is immediately noticeable, look into it. In Figure 8.1 the pigment at 12 o'clock stands out and should be explored for its potential significance,

especially since it also coincides with another sign: a large lacuna, in the same location.

2. Several signs point to the same organ or system—e.g., small signs in the liver reflex site, yellow or brown pigmentation (topolabile) in other sectors, and pupil flattening adjacent to the liver sector. In this case, whatever the symptoms, you will probably benefit from looking after your liver. In the iris in Figure 8.2, the lacunae situated on pancreatic reflex zones are amplified by the scattered orange "pancreotropic" pigments: both sets of signs portend issues with sustaining stable blood sugar levels.

3. Contrasting signs appear in the same organ sector—e.g., bright signs combined with dark signs, such as a deep lacuna bordered by bright white fibers (perifocal brightness). This shows an area where there may be some conflict, with possibly painful consequences. The bright sign denotes high reactivity, and the dark sign tells you that there is a core of negativity and possible degeneration. The likelihood of symptoms arising in such an area is high. Another example is a lacuna and a pigment appearing in the same location: these signs have opposite meanings, therefore there may be an "energetic conflict." In Figure 8.3, several deep crypts are encircled by thick, bright white fibrous borders, highlighting possible areas of chronic inflammation. Note also the dark and bright patches within the stomach zone.

Also note appearances that suggest problems that may be latent or undiscovered, such as a lipemic or cholesterol ring, which can point to a potentially life-threatening blood condition. Anchor your observations to what is verifiable; for example, if you see a lipemic ring, you can consider taking a cholesterol test, if you see signs suggestive of blood sugar problems you can test for that, and so forth. I am not, by the way, recommending that you test for every possibility that you see; however, if for example you have a strong family history in that department, and you also have a suggestive iris sign, it would be doing due diligence for your own health to keep an eye on the markers.

You also can start to make deductions from your symptoms and case history about the presence of signs. For example, if you

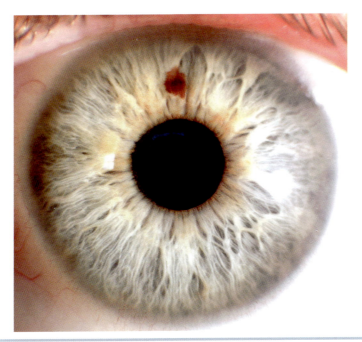

FIGURE 8.1

A sign that stands out at 12 o'clock.

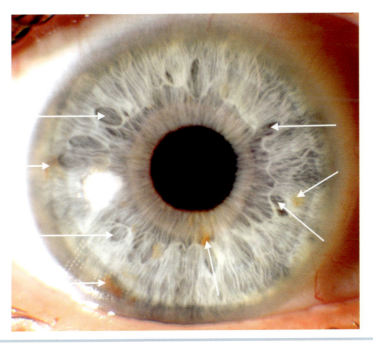

FIGURE 8.2

Lacunae on pancreatic reflex zones and scattered orange "pancreotropic" pigments.

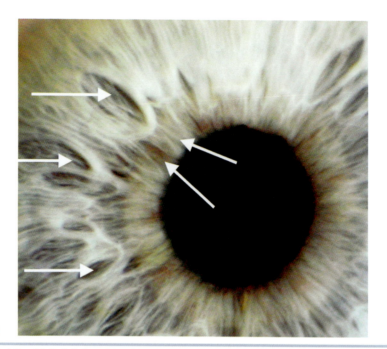

FIGURE 8.3

Crypts encircled by thick, bright white fibrous borders.

suffered from childhood eczema and have rough irritable skin as an adult, you will want to check to see if you have a scurf rim circling your iris. If you do, you can further deduce that you are having difficulty eliminating toxins and waste products, and you can examine other organs and systems concerned with elimination. From this assessment, you can begin to identify possible causes for the problems you are experiencing (e.g., stress, liver function, kidney strength).

Deviations from circularity

Observing the circular structures of the irides—the pupillary ruff or pupil margin, the collarette, contraction furrows, and the circularity of the iris itself—can give you information about your nervous system. Occasionally, the iris is not completely circular, and this may mean that the neuromuscular system could be a factor in any problems you are experiencing. Sometimes the disturbance in circularity is obvious. In Figure 8.4 there is a flattening of the iris in the lower segment, but also in the upper sections relating to neck and upper thoracic spine. This person was suffering from extreme pain as a result of rigidity of the lumbar spine, which was relieved by means of osteopathic adjustment. However, there remained a tendency for the same pattern to recur under stress, so work on the upper part of the spine is also needed to clear the imbalance.

Nerve supply problems to the organs may also be important factors to assess, and are suggested by patterns of flattening around the pupil ring, as well as by indentations or jaggedness of the collarette.

Density and resistance

Density is a measure of resistance. (For a discussion of the overall density of iris fiber structure, see discussion of the structural types in Chapter 4.) In general, the denser your iris, the more resistant you are, and the less dense, the less resistant you are. It is important

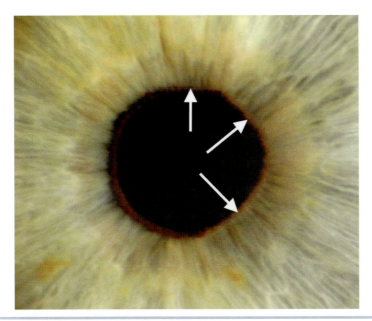

FIGURE 8.4

Disturbances of spinal alignment shown by flatness in the upper and lower sectors of the pupil margin.

to know your level of resistance in order to make appropriate adjustments to your lifestyle as part of any treatment plan. Also, in assessing the impact of stress, your degree of tolerance must be taken into consideration. Your lifestyle may be putting undue strain on your constitution if it is delicate. The measure of resistance in individual organs is also important. Note areas of reduced fiber density that may alert you to specific organ problems. Low resistance in any area may be seen in features such as lacunae and rarefaction, or a loosening of the texture of the iris.

Shading

This refers to dark or light appearances in the iris, which give information about the ability of your system or of an individual organ to react. Whiteness or brightness shows high reactivity, with a tendency to inflammation and acute symptoms; dark and black areas suggest an absence of reactivity, with the danger of failure to act in defense against illnesses and harmful influences, resulting over time in potential tissue degeneration and destruction. A dark iris shows a system that may not be able to react sufficiently to protect itself. A bright, pale iris with whiteness may tend toward overreactivity and chronic inflammation—the rheumatic iris type.

Assessing individual organs for their ability to react or not, and whether there is a tendency to chronic over- or underreactivity, can be important. For example, if your iris has a loose texture and dark shading in the kidney sector and you have skin problems, one factor in your condition may be underfunctioning of the kidneys, which would also be a clue to resolving the problem.

ASSESSING FAMILIAL TRAITS

If, when assessing significant signs, you come across something that seems to be important, yet which is not in your case history, it may suggest familial traits. Consider whether anyone in your family has suffered with the problem indicated. Check whether there is any arthritis, high blood pressure, diabetes, heart weakness, or bowel

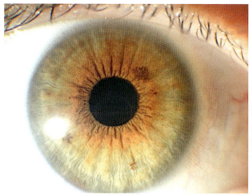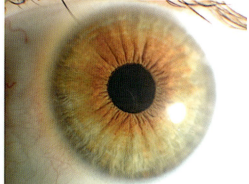

FIGURE 8.5

Paternal genetic dominance shown by the presence of secondary pigments in the right iris, but not in the left.

problems, etc., in your family. In many cases, health problems experienced by your parents or grandparents may be lying in wait for you as you grow older, and conditions such as some types of breast cancer clearly may run genetically through the female line of a family. You also need to assess how likely it is that a problem that seems to be indicated in your iris will actually occur. It is possible that a sign may reflect a family condition that has not surfaced for generations.

How important are these traits when assessing your own health risks or predispositions? If your mother had high blood pressure does that mean you will have the same problem? Bearing in mind that different traits come through different lines of the family, can we predict the inherited elements that we may manifest?

The two distinct strands that make up your inheritance are visible in your irides; the right iris relates chiefly to paternal inheritance, the left to maternal. The iris with the most prominent structural signs, or the highest number of signs, is the dominant iris. If structure is not conclusive, look at pigments as well.

In Figure 8.5 we see the irides of a person whose dominant genetic influence is paternal—note secondary pigments in the right iris but not the left. Your eyes may not show such an obvious variation, but if you can determine which iris is dominant, it is a clue as to which of your parents has passed your main health predispositions down to you, and what health threats may most affect you.

SUMMARY OF IRIS ANALYSIS

1. Note any current symptoms.
2. Record your case history.
3. Observe your iris display, noting the following information:
    a. *Color:* three basic types
    b. *Structure/texture:* five basic types
    c. *Overlay:* four basic types
4. *Signs:* Note three to five signs that either pervade (e.g., cholesterol ring, hyperacidic clouding) or that stand out in the iris (e.g., a large lacuna, pigment spot, or central heterochromia).
5. Perform a basic crosscheck between symptoms (past and present) and iris indications.
6. If the crosscheck is negative, consider the possible contribution of vital organs—such as the liver and kidneys—to your symptoms.
7. Consider how your iris display may reflect your family history, where known. If necessary, assess which iris is dominant, that is, the probability of characteristics being passed down from one parent.
8. Construct a three- or four-point health plan that covers your basic indications and helps to prevent the main risks to your health, using the suggestions in Chapters 3 to 5.

For example, if you have a lymphatic constitution and a high-resistance structure with a hyperacidic overlay, you will need to pay attention to elimination, detoxification, and immunity. You will also need to consider what you can do to balance and nourish your nervous system and pay specific attention to eliminating acids from your body. You also can adopt a diet that will help to minimize acid formation.

If you have a hematogenic constitution, self-protective structure, and lipemic overlay, blood cleansing will be important to keep your blood composition healthy; cayenne and ginger will help to stimulate your circulation; nerve treatments and muscle relaxants will treat your tendency for cramping and nervous tension; and treating your liver will assist in bringing blood fats down to normal levels. In addition, you need to make efforts to clear accumulated fats out of the circulatory vessels.

DRAWING A BLANK

What do you do if your assessment doesn't make sense, when you see signs that indicate problems that you don't seem to have, when nothing seems to match up, and you do not recognize yourself in your assessment? There are a few reasons why this might happen:

▹ The indications are latent tendencies and have not yet manifested. When a problem is likely to appear is different for each person depending a lot on lifestyle and individual stressors.

▹ A symptom is a warning that your constitutional tolerances have been breached. If you live in a way that supports your weak points and avoids threats, the symptom may not appear at all. Severe problems in the past may be clearly reflected in your iris display, even though you are now free from discomfort through having made the necessary adjustments.

▹ You are not ready to become conscious of yourself in this way or you may not want to face the problems. High-resistance type people sometimes find it hard to admit that there may be good cause to change their lifestyles, and they also seem to be able to absorb a lot of stress.

▹ You are seeing factors that influence the general environment of the body. We do not generally *feel* liver congestion, yet when it is a factor, other things may start to malfunction. This is the less immediately verifiable aspect of iridology that works with the concept of the prepathological—the slight disturbances of homeostasis or metabolic function that may eventually add up to something more serious. In this case, there is work to be done on a preventive level. (See Chapter 10.)

> ‣ The indications are emotionally or psychologically significant, rather than physically. Guidance will be given on this possibility in a later book.

At any rate, you are now ready to go out and try your skills. Make sure, if you use others as your "guinea pigs," that you tell them that you are not professionally qualified, and do refer to a professional in the case of anyone presenting with worrying symptoms, or where problems are suggested in the iris that are beyond your knowledge level.

When conducting iris investigations on friends and family, I strongly suggest you have this book handy in case you need to find answers to any questions that arise, and also a copy of the iris topography chart (Figure 6.13).

9

Iris portraits
and specific conditions

An iris portrait is a collection of iris indicators that point to a particular problem. It is not a hard-and-fast diagnosis; it simply means that there is a high chance of the suggested health problem manifesting. Iris indications also flag up abnormalities or possible system deficiencies that, over a period of time, may bring about a certain condition. By the onset of an identifiable disease, there have usually been many years of pre- or subclinical events. The limits of tolerance in one's system, the requirements of homeostasis, are quite narrow. Homeostasis may be described as the process by which the internal systems of the body—pressure, temperature, acid–alkaline balance, and so on—are maintained in equilibrium, despite variations in external conditions.

The following sections list the kinds of appearances that suggest possible problems. The principles are *energetic* in nature—we look to see if an organ is over- or underactive; or showing deficiency or excess. Remember that white equals overreactive, dark equals underreactive; loose equals low resistance, tight equals high resistance; lacunae equals emptiness and deficiency; pigment equals fullness and excess.

ARTHRITIS AND RHEUMATISM

The definition of *acute* inflammation is the local response to cellular injury. In this context the word "injury" refers to anything that damages or kills cells, which is automatically met by a cascade of biochemical and functional changes whose aim is to clear away the injurious agent, protect against further damage, and then repair and remodel the tissue—which is called *resolution.* It is a very basic function of our *immunity.*

When acute inflammation fails to be "switched off" by the body, this may be taken to indicate that the injurious agent, or something perceived by the body to be injurious, has not been successfully removed and is still stimulating this attempt at resolution. This is referred to as *chronic* inflammation—chronic simply meaning long-lasting.

Arthritis and rheumatism are examples of chronic inflammation. They show an ongoing attempt by your body to isolate and resolve a long-standing problem. Our task as healers is to identify the underlying cause and help the body to remove it, and in this the iris display can usefully assist in presenting us with factors that may be involved: a hyperacidic overlay, for example, refers to the abnormal retention of acidic wastes; failure or suboptimal function of organs of detoxification and elimination—bowel, kidneys, liver, and lymph—leading to accumulations of pathogenic materials (chemicals and heavy metals, for example). Enzyme deficiencies (the dyscratic overlay) may be slowing down the body's natural mechanisms for breaking down and removing foreign matter.

This is the way we "translate" iris information into naturopathic intervention: we don't simply look for the nearest "anti-inflammatory" herb or supplement (though these may have a temporary benefit in relieving unbearable pain): we get going on what needs to be done—alkalizing the system through appropriate diet and digestive upgrades, activating the organs of secretion and elimination so that we start to get ahead of accumulating levels of toxins and impurities that are affecting our immune response.

There are more than a hundred variations of arthritis, medically speaking; however, the main types are osteoarthritis (OA) and rheumatoid arthritis (RA). The latter is considered to have an autoimmune component (the immune system "attacks" the body), while the former, far more common, is often described as "wear and tear," and 80% of the over-65-year-old population has radiographic evidence of OA. However, chronically, a complication of rheumatoid arthritis is osteoarthritis (inflammation-mediated destruction of cartilage), and the proinflammatory mechanisms involved in osteoarthritis, even if they are not themselves officially "autoimmune," have a similar tendency to progressively involve the surrounding tissue structures and cause much collateral damage.

Iris signs do not really distinguish between different types of arthritis. While it is sometimes possible to point to a predisposition to arthritis, it is not usually possible to say which kind. It is fortunate, therefore, that the naturopathic and herbal interventions that are effective at treating these conditions will generally work for both types.

Relevant iris signs

White arc at the iris border: A white frosted arc at the margin of the iris (usually the nasal aspect) is known as a *spondalarthritic arc*. Such a white arc indicates high risk for osteoarthritis (Figure 9.1); it is also considered to point to a family history of tuberculosis. The dyscratic overlay in this iris is an additional risk factor.

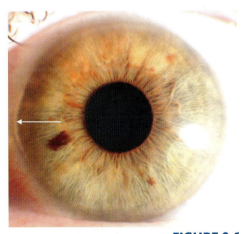

FIGURE 9.1

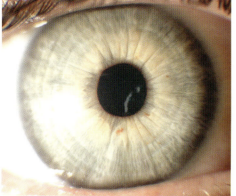

FIGURE 9.2

Bright white fibers: These indicate a rheumatic iris (Figure 9.2). In a pale lymphatic (blue-eyed) type person, the overall impression of whiteness may also be caused by the presence of a neurogenic disposition, where the fibers are pressed close together, so the reflective property of the stroma is amplified. In this case there will also be involvement of nerves and stress.

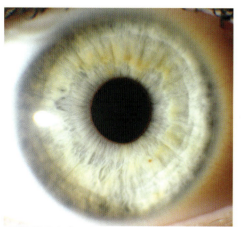

FIGURE 9.3

White or pale yellow cloudy plaques: White or pale yellow cloudy plaques or wisps in the ciliary zone (the hyperacidic overlay) suggest a "urinary" type, with high levels of uric acid in the tissues(Figure 9.3). The yellow tinge may indicate impaired kidney function and a toxic bowel; there is also a risk for all forms of arthritis, especially gout.

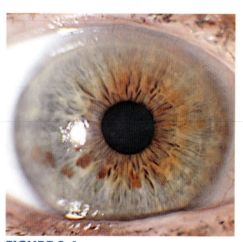

FIGURE 9.4

The dyscratic overlay: multiple pigment patches suggest enzyme deficiency and reduced detoxification potential; this type has soft tissue rheumatic disease as a listed risk factor (Figure 9.4).[1]

Light mixed type with cloudy overlay: General cloudiness of the ciliary zone suggests poor resolution of acid wastes. In brown eyes, particularly of the mixed type, the tendency towards sluggish digestion might also contribute to the level of risk (Figure 9.5).

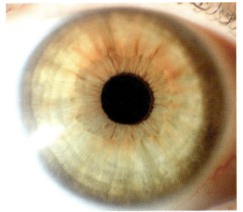

FIGURE 9.5

Transversal fibers: Fibers running across the grain through the fourth minor zone—the spinal reflex area (musculoskeletal zone)—indicate irritation and inflammation (Figure 9.6).

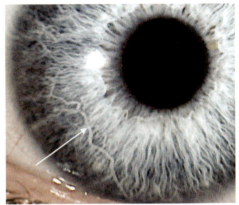

FIGURE 9.6

Pupil flatness: Disturbed circularity of the iris may indicate rigidity or misalignment in the spinal system (Figure 9.7).

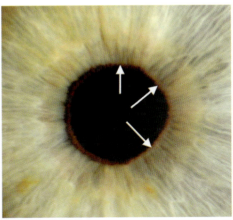

FIGURE 9.7

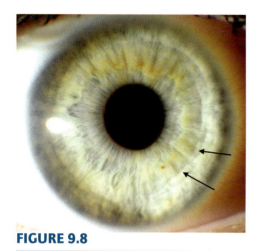

FIGURE 9.8

Contraction furrows: Circular furrows, with some fragmentation, running through the spinal reflex zone, and other signs affecting the ciliary zone reflexes for the spine and cervical spine, indicate that neuromuscular tension may be driving arthritic inflammation (Figure 9.8).

A portrait for arthritic risk factors

In Figure 9.9 we see yellowish cloudy plaques, giving the iris an overall greenish appearance. The dark color inside the central ring, the pupillary zone or collarette, suggests low stomach acid, sluggishness of the bowel, and retention of toxic wastes that may be reabsorbed by the body, placing stress on the kidneys and leading to reabsorption of acidic wastes, a potential cause of inflammation. The dark outer band (scurf rim) suggests difficulties with the elimination of acidic waste products. Note also the slight flattening of the iris at the lower left margin, indicating possible problems with the lumbar spine, and patterns of flatness in the upper right pupil margin, denoting possible neck problems. There are also circular furrows running through the fourth minor zone in Figure 9.9. Areas of stress and tension affecting the musculoskeletal system increase the risk of arthritic development in that location.

Suggested remedies

Diet: The famous American herbalist John R. Christopher taught that arthritis of any kind was at least partly caused by dietary error, citing "mucus-forming foods" as the main culprits.[2] Staying away from the usual suspects ("white" carbs including sugar, dairy produce, caffeine, and alcohol) and maximizing fresh produce (fruits and vegetables) is highly beneficial. (See also Paavo Airola's book, *There Is a Cure for Arthritis*.[3]) In addition, many practitioners feel that foods derived from the nightshade family, the *Solonaceae*—potatoes, tomatoes, eggplant (aubergine), and peppers—significantly aggravate a tendency to arthritis.

Detoxification: Perform a full program of detox routines on a regular basis to offset the deficit in removal of acidic wastes (see Chapter 10).

Hydrotherapy: Alternate hot and cold showers, saunas, and steam rooms (with cold plunges), sitz baths, alternating hot and cold external packs. Also apply hydrotherapy locally, ending with

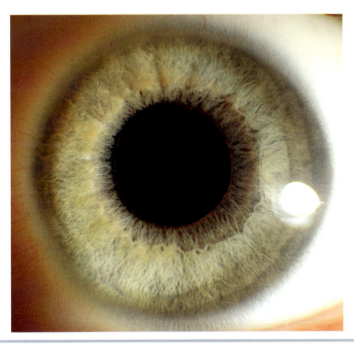

FIGURE 9.9

Yellowish cloudy plaques (hyperacidic type)
with dark inner and outer zones.

hot water in the first stages of treatment (see Chapter 10). After performing this, use a "deep heat" topical ointment, rubbing it into the affected area to improve circulation and help rebuild tissues.

Topical oil or ointment: To make your own oil, cover equal parts by weight of grated ginger root, chopped cayenne pods, St John's wort herb, arnica flowers, and calendula flowers with a good organic cold-pressed olive oil for two weeks, shaking the mixture twice daily. Strain the herbs and add essential oils of peppermint wintergreen (a 50|ml bottle should contain around 15–20 drops of each oil).

Exercise: Although problematic for people with arthritic pain, it is necessary to persevere with exercise to keep your circulation active and your joints supple. Swimming is ideal, as skeletal shock and weight-bearing is reduced though the support of water. Gentle Hatha Yoga can also be beneficial.

Herbal choices

Celery seed, dandelion leaf, nettle herb (to assist in removal of acidic wastes); bogbean, devil's claw, frankincense, turmeric (inflammation-modulating); wild lettuce, valerian, Jamaican dogwood, black cohosh, wild yam (for pain relief); ginger, cayenne, mustard seed, prickly ash bark (to promote circulation).

A case of arthritis

Joanne was 36 years old and had a diagnosis of psoriatic arthritis with symptoms of lupus. Both these conditions are chronic inflammatory connective tissue complaints with an autoimmune element.

Arthritis had come on quickly with little warning, affecting many of her joints to some extent, but especially her knees. Her doctor wanted to give her immunosuppressant drugs, and she had been given a steroid to help control the inflammation, together

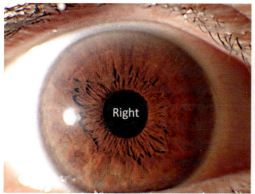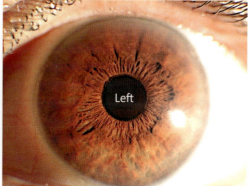

FIGURE 9.10

Joanne.

with a three-times-a-day dose of aspirin, none of which she wanted to take long-term.

Joanne also suffered from poor circulation and chilblains, felt tired and listless, suffered occasional irritable bowel symptoms, and did not sleep well. Her immunity generally was low, and she became highly susceptible to viral infections.

Although she followed a vegetarian diet, Joanne relied heavily on sugar, refined carbohydrate products, French fries, and dairy products. She drank more than eight cups of tea or coffee daily (with two teaspoons of sugar), and she craved acidic foods such as tomatoes and vinegar—all contraindicated in her condition— and chocolate, especially at the time of menstruation. She did no exercise.

Irides

Joanne's color type is dark mixed, showing a typical pattern of a darker nutritive zone and collarette, and a ciliary zone with lighter, greenish patches (Figure 9.10). Darker pigment patches at 8 minutes left and 38 minutes right in the ciliary zone are suggestive of reduced liver detoxification. The iris structure is gastric, with lacunae and crypts inside the collarette. There are the beginnings of a lipemic (cholesterol) ring in the upper sector (blood stagnation), and the presence of a spondalarthritic arc at the inner margins of each iris.

Indentations of the collarette border in both irides at 6 o'clock suggest pressure on adrenals and susceptibility to stress. The prominent, rope-like appearance of the collarette around much of its length suggests nervous irritability of digestion and bowel. There are honeycombs (collections of crypts) in various locations in the digestive reflex areas of both irides, suggestive of dysbiosis—a big driver of autoimmune inflammation—and possible parasitic infestation.

Treatment

Joanne reformed her diet radically, eliminating tea, coffee, sugar, and the saturated and highly heated fats in the dairy products and fried foods. This relieved pressure on her liver and digestion. She also cut out nightshade foods—tomatoes, potatoes, peppers, and eggplant.

She ate more fresh fruit and vegetables, drank plenty of filtered water, and took an individually prepared herbal formula, which included blood purifiers (nettle and yellow dock), a digestive bitter (gentian root), antirheumatics (devil's claw and meadowsweet), antispasmodics (black cohosh and skullcap), and a circulatory stimulant (ginger). She also paid attention to her stress levels and became aware of when her body warned that she was exceeding her limits of tolerance through joint pains and skin outbreaks.

Three weeks after her first visit, the improvements were dramatic. The first time she had visited, she had to be seen in a downstairs office as she could not manage the stairs. On her first follow-up visit she breezed in, bounded past me, and virtually sprang up the stairs.

Her treatment continued, with a full bowel and liver cleanse, the application of hydrotherapy on affected joints, and gentle exercise to stretch out the ligaments.

She continued to suffer with symptoms from time to time, especially under stress, but she knew what triggered her condition and how to make changes to her lifestyle where and when necessary.

THE GASTROINTESTINAL TRACT

The iris is a particularly good guide for assessing digestion. Our digestive systems are active almost constantly, and in these days of high-stress living, comfort eating, poor quality food, and other toxic influences and habits, they are under siege. The correct operation of the digestive tract is fundamental to all other organs and systems. Its malfunction is a factor in a range of complaints.

Indigestion, acid stomach, and reflux

In classical iridology, excess stomach acidity, indigestion, and esophageal reflux are all suggested by a bright white stomach halo. This implies overactivity of the stomach, with excess production of hydrochloric acid. Reflux is said to be the result when this acid escapes upward into the esophagus, particularly when the valve at the top end of the stomach is weak or damaged. This weakness can be exacerbated through overeating or by eating too many acid-forming foods. The resulting symptoms will disappear once eating habits have been corrected.

However, it is far more common (see "The Mixed Biliary Constitution," Chapter 3) that we see undersecretion of stomach acid—hypochlorhydria—which would be indicated by a dark gray color affecting the stomach ring. In this case there will be delayed gastric emptying, with the risk of upward regurgitation specifically linked to epigastric fullness and bloating. There may also be weakness of the lower esophageal sphincter. (See "The Digestive System," in Chapter 6.)

Treatment

Treatment for indigestion, acid stomach, and reflux includes practicing mealtime hygiene (see "The Mixed Biliary Constitution," in Chapter 3), reducing acid-forming foods, and, particularly, reducing intake of refined wheat products and dairy products.

Herbal choices

Slippery elm, marshmallow, and licorice powders in drinks will absorb acids and heal and regenerate the stomach lining. Herbs taken as teas or tinctures such as meadowsweet and dandelion normalize stomach secretions, while centaury herb strengthens a weakened lower esophageal sphincter.

Food sensitivity and irritable bowel syndrome

If you have digestive pain or discomfort, the food that you eat may be the cause; however, the *way you eat* must also be subject to scrutiny. The incidence of food allergy or intolerance is high and getting higher: is it simply down to endemic poor food choices, or does the pressure of life itself perhaps have a role to play?

Sensitivity reactions involving foods may, however, be suspected wherever you see brightness and reactivity of the collarette. If you have a hyperreactive or allergic tendency, there may be reactivity in your gastrointestinal tract, with the accompanying symptoms of griping pain and spasm, alternating constipation and diarrhea, and bloating and distension of the abdomen. This complex of symptoms is often called "irritable bowel syndrome" (IBS). The nerves and stress are frequently involved, as is the failure to break down foods adequately in the upper reaches of the digestive tract. It is potentially a complex syndrome, and sometimes the exclusion of foods that are assumed to be troublesome does nothing in particular except cause the system to find other foods to react to! This can lead to ever more restrictive diets and even, potentially, to malnutrition.

There is a famous saying in Ayurveda: "When digestive fire is strong, you can turn poison into nectar." We may gather from this that the baseline of good digestion is to be sought in the secretory powers of the stomach, the liver and gallbladder, and the pancreas. When addressing so-called "food sensitivities" (or even allergies or intolerances), it is vital to bear this in mind.

Food sensitivities may be involved in other symptoms; temporarily excluding the "offending" foods may relieve other allergic tendencies, such as hay fever and asthma, as well as general fatigue, reduced mental function, and depression. Sensitivity to otherwise healthy foods might also be improved by a period of recuperation, where reducing aggravating influences such as stress and unhealthy food in order to rest will strengthen and rebuild the digestive system.

Iris signs

Hypersensitivity of the gastrointestinal tract is seen most often in blue-eyed people, because of their generally heightened reactivity; but a prominent, ropy, or jagged collarette may indicate this tendency in people of any eye color. Strong coloring of the collarette can add to the diagnosis. In Figure 9.11, note not only the prominence of the collarette, but also the strong yellow pigmentation. This indicates involvement of the liver/gallbladder, and a high probability of sensitivity to or intolerance of dairy fats.

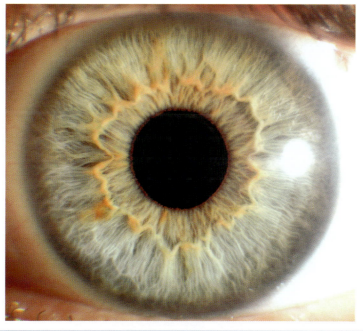

FIGURE 9.11

Prominent (hypertonic) collarette border with yellow pigmentation.

Treatment

Treatment for food sensitivity and irritable bowel syndrome includes identifying possible allergens, such as dairy foods, wheat, and yeast.

People suffering from these problems should try to reduce their stress levels and practice strict mealtime hygiene. The hematogenic iris with a hypertonic "rope-like" collarette border in Figure 9.12 would have similar tendencies toward irritable bowel and food sensitivities.

Herbal choices

Herbs can be taken as teas or tinctures, to treat nerves: skullcap, passionflower, or valerian. Antispasmodic herbs that can be used include wild yam, black cohosh, and peppermint. Practicing food combining and taking bitter tonics will promote better digestion, thus minimizing potentially aggravating matter entering the colon. Pau d'arco, barberry root bark, black walnut hulls, and wormwood improve gastrointestinal immunity and control candida.

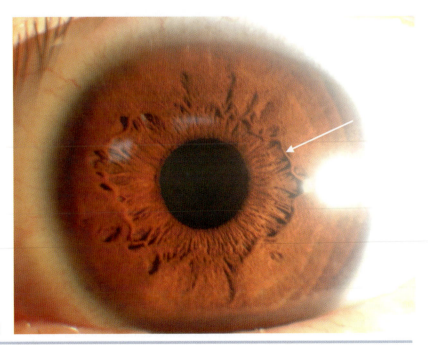

FIGURE 9.12

Hematogenic iris showing a hypertonic "rope-like" collarette border.

A case of Crohn's disease

Crohn's disease (CD) is an autoimmune inflammatory condition—one of the two main pathologies that come under the inflammatory bowel disease heading.

Michael was 45 years old when he first came to see me; he had had Crohn's disease since the age of 17. In that time, he had had two periods of remission, the last one 6 years previously, but he had a severe relapse a year before his visit to me.

Crohn's can affect any part of the digestive tract from mouth to anus, but Michael's trouble area was the lower end of the colon—the sigmoid colon and rectum. He was experiencing up to 15 bowel movements daily, with blood and pus. Pain and abdominal cramps would start shortly after eating; he was constantly fatigued and suffered with greatly reduced cognitive functions—memory and concentration.

Medical treatments included a mild anti-inflammatory, prednisolone (a steroid medication), and a very strong antibiotic, metronidazole.

Lifestyle and diet

Michael did no exercise, as it brought on attacks. He commuted to work in London, where he held down a high-powered job in the corporate sector. His diet relied heavily on refined carbohydrates, but when I saw him, he had already given up coffee (which helped a great deal), dairy produce, and other greasy, fatty foods, and had started to take fish oils, which he also found beneficial. He did, however, still drink around half a bottle of red wine every other evening; he reported that he used to be far less moderate in the past.

Irides

Michael's irides are unusual in that the color classification is extremely individual (Figure 9.13). They are somewhere between a lymphatic dyscratic and a mixed biliary hydrogenoid. The most unusual feature is the very strong orange coloring in the various spots and plaques, in both the central ring and the peripheral

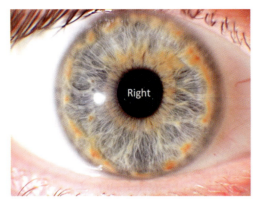 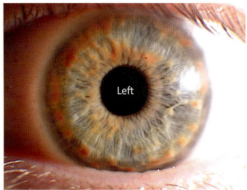

FIGURE 9.13

Michael.

lymph rosary. The bright orange color suggests pancreatic imbalance, with consequent risks for poor breakdown and absorption and blood sugar irregularities.

The most interesting feature regarding the presenting condition is in the reflex to the descending and sigmoid colon, where we not only see distension of the collarette, with loose tissue locally (a version of the gastric disposition), but also five very clearly defined "tophi," like a mini lymph rosary on the collarette border, involving the gut-associated lymphatic tissue—affecting gastrointestinal immunity. These spots are also quite bright, suggesting a high level of reactivity—with inflammation right on site where we would expect to see it, in the lower end of the colon.

Treatment

My initial recommendations included cutting out wheat products, maintaining a predominantly plant-based diet, the immediate exclusion of all caffeine and alcohol, and the introduction of mild stretching exercises. All of this he readily took on.

I gave herbal powders of slippery elm bark, marshmallow root, licorice root, bayberry bark, and golden seal root, to take three times daily away from food (mid-morning, mid-afternoon, before sleep), and a herbal tincture aimed at balancing immunity, controlling pathogens in the gut, astringing the intestinal walls to stop undue discharge, and a deep cleanse for the lymphatic system.

Within one week Michael experienced a 70% improvement: less frequent bowel motions, with no griping or pain. Within two weeks this had progressed to a 90% improvement, and bowel motions were down to 3 or 4 daily.

Subsequent visits to a gastroenterologist revealed substantial histological improvements and enabled a reduction in drug doses. Over time flare-ups became less frequent and less severe; eventually all drugs were stopped. Michael has been in remission now for a few years. He still uses herbs to maintain optimal digestive and immune function.

Sluggish digestion

People with a mixed iris type often have signs that show a more sluggish digestive system; however, the presence of additional pigmentation over the digestive zone in any iris will tend to suggest similar conditions, with epigastric discomfort or pain experienced shortly after eating—a feeling of tightness and distension around the midriff. Bloating can tend to get worse as the day goes on, and eating too late is likely to exacerbate the problem.

Iris signs

Figure 9.14 shows a blue eye with an orange central heterochromia. The individual suffered from severe bloating whenever she ate. A dark nutritive zone, with perhaps a tinge of brown/gray, can also suggest sluggishness of digestion through low gastric acid provision and associated dysbiosis.

Treatment

A sluggish digestion can be resolved not only with changes in the individual's diet, but also by taking herbal bitters, which stimulate the secretion of digestive fluids from the liver, gallbladder, and pancreas. Food-combining principles (see Chapter 10) were included in the recommendations. Taking care not to overload the digestive system with unsuitable combinations of foods protects the organs of secretion and extends their functional life. For this

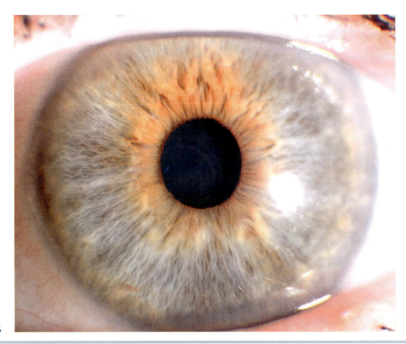

FIGURE 9.14

Orange central heterochromia.

reason also we generally do not recommend the once-popular practice of eating little and often to help sustain blood sugar levels: this likewise places extra pressure on the pancreas, in particular.

Spasmodic disorders

As we have seen, the nervous system plays a large part in the health of the gastrointestinal tract, and people of the self-protective type (see Chapter 4) are particularly predisposed to gastrointestinal spasms. This can be seen in the radial furrows, sometimes called "spasm furrows," in the iris.

Iris signs

Radial furrows show high levels of gastrointestinal stress, and are associated with cramping and spasmodic pain in the gut. Major

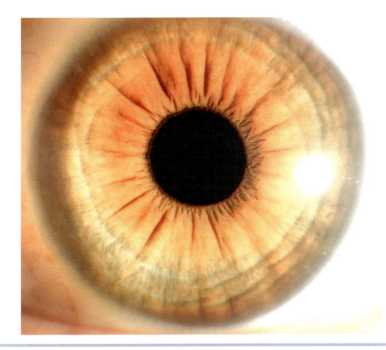

FIGURE 9.15

This mixed biliary larvate tetanic iris shows multiple radials (*spasm furrows*) impacting on the digestive zone.

radials also are seen to cut through the collarette and may weaken the nerve supply for digestion. In the iris shown in Figure 9.15 the collarette is extremely contracted toward the pupil in a "drawstring" effect, also implying poor gastrointestinal dynamics and spasms. Note also the degree of contraction of the collarette border.

Herbal choices

Recommended herbs include wild yam and cramp bark, best taken as tinctures.

Constipation

There are a few possible causes of constipation, and the iris may be useful in determining the exact cause. For example, two opposite types of constipation are *spastic* and *atonal*, and they need different treatments. With spastic constipation, the emphasis is on releasing and relaxation. With atonal constipation, the peristaltic muscles must be activated.

Constipation may also occur through insufficient secretion of bile from the liver/gallbladder, or through lack of hydration. In cases where bile secretion is thought to be low, drinking a full glass of water approximately 30 minutes before each meal and then taking a few drops of a bitter tonic tincture just before the meal could be helpful.

The ideal frequency of bowel movement is one motion about 20 minutes after each meal. This may prove difficult to achieve and sustain, but once managed, you will be in no doubt of the benefits. If you think about it, if you are eating three times a day but only evacuating once a day or less, there is a clear risk of unwanted retention, and any amount of retention is a threat to optimum health.

Iris signs

Spastic constipation is suggested by a tightly contracted collarette and radial furrows. Atonal constipation, where peristaltic muscles are flaccid and unresponsive, appears as distension of the collarette, possibly with lacunae or crypts in the nutritive zone, as in the Gastric disposition (see chapter 4). Liver-related signs can indicate a problem with bile secretion—adequate secretion of bile is a strong necessity for good bowel function.

Herbal choices

Herbs to relieve constipation include senna, cascara, and aloe, best taken in capsules (for atonal constipation); linseeds, psyllium husk, slippery elm powder, and licorice powders mixed into water act as bulking laxatives; wild yam and black cohosh taken as tinctures help a spastic colon, IBS, and diverticulitis; gentian, barberry, wormwood, and bitter herbs promote bile production. Adequate hydration is of great importance in every case.

THE HORMONE SYSTEM

The hormone system is one of the body's two important messenger networks, the other being the nervous system. The hormonal organs are all interconnected in a unified system that is largely controlled by the master gland in the brain, the pituitary, which sends triggering hormones throughout the body to stimulate and regulate the activity of the other endocrine glands.

Hypoglycemia/diabetes

Iris signs

A tendency to diabetes/hypoglycemia is indicated by any combination of the following factors:

- the hormone-regulatory structural type;
- leaf-shaped lacuna at 4 o'clock in the left iris (pancreas tail);
- shiny orange pigments anywhere in either iris;
- square shape of the collarette;
- violet hue inside the collarette (nutritive zone);
- hematogenic constitution;
- lipemic overlay (there is a close connection between high blood fats and diabetes).

Figure 9.16, of a left iris, belongs to a young patient with pronounced blood sugar problems. Note the lacunae at around 10 minutes and 20 minutes, and the overall square-ish appearance of the collarette border. Also note the patchy orange (pancreotropic) pigment at 22 minutes. In such a case, ask about family history of Type 2 diabetes, and individual symptoms of hypoglycemia: becoming hungry suddenly, with feelings of faintness, nausea, or irritation ("hangry"). There may also be general cravings for sweet things and refined carbohydrates.

This illustrates an important principle in focusing on individual signs: where several different signs point to the same diagnosis, we should always pay attention.

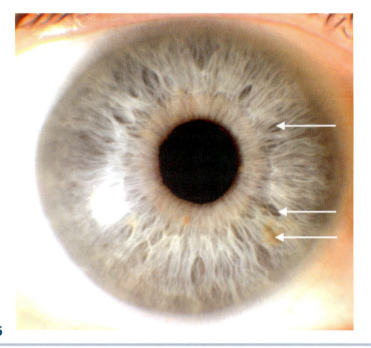

FIGURE 9.16

Left iris, of a young patient with pronounced blood sugar problems.

Treatment

In traditional medicine this condition goes hand in hand with digestive weakness, so digestion should always be treated alongside any other specific concerns. Practicing appropriate mealtime hygiene and using digestive stimulants in the diet, or as specific medicines, will be effective.

Diet: Reduce intake of refined sugars and carbohydrates.

Herbal choices

For digestion: Bitter tonics: gentian root, centaury herb, wormwood herb, barberry root bark.

To normalize blood sugar: Burdock, Siberian ginseng, neem, goat's rue, garlic, fenugreek.

To reduce sugar cravings: Gymnema.

The female hormone system

This system is closely connected with the other endocrine organs; for example, many women become hypoglycemic at the time of menstruation. Also, women need strong adrenals during the menopause, because when the ovaries stop producing estrogen, the adrenals take over to supplement the drop in output up to around 25%. Women who avoid excessive stress and take adrenal-boosting herbs such as Siberian ginseng, astragalus, and licorice are likely to have an easier menopause.

The appearance of signs in the pituitary and adrenal zones is particularly important when assessing the health of the menstrual cycle. The pituitary, in particular, as the master hormone gland, is responsible for the signals that ensure menstruation happens on schedule, and that the fertility cycle is operating as it should.

A case of dysmenorrhea

The irides shown in Figure 9.17 are those of a young woman of only 15 who was experiencing difficulties with her periods right from the beginning, at the age of 14; this included erratic cycles, severe PMS, and painful cramps and spasms.

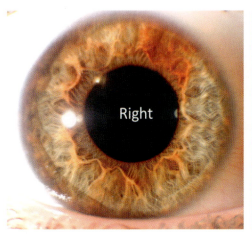
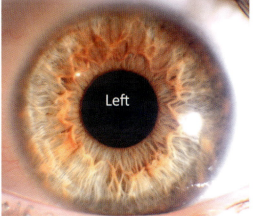

FIGURE 9.17

April.

The constitution is mixed biliary hormone-regulatory—always remember, whenever treating hormones, that digestion may be crucial. In this case the strong orange color denotes a particular focus on the pancreas and blood sugar; she also experienced strong sugar cravings at the time of the month.

Note in the left iris the crypts at 12 o'clock and 6 o'clock, pituitary and adrenal, suggesting the role of stress in the overall symptom picture. In the right iris, note in the lower sector a structural disturbance of the whole "kidney" area, with a break in the collarette and rarefaction in the uterus reflex zone.

Treatment

Asking a patient to make far-reaching dietary changes when she is already feeling disturbed and uncomfortable is probably going to be unproductive, so it was important to provide some stability for this young woman as a sign of good faith! Fortunately, there are some extremely effective and powerful herbal assistants for these issues, and these were given in a formula that consisted of Dong Quai (regulates hormones via the pituitary gland), black cohosh (antispasmodic for menstrual cramps), dandelion root (to optimize the metabolization of excess estrogen in the liver), mugwort (a wonderful herb that combines antispasmodic emmenagogue properties with digestion-promoting actions), motherwort (a calming and nurturing herb that also has strong affinities with the female reproductive system), and rose (liver-cleansing, hormone-harmonizing and all-round mood enhancer).

When treating the female hormonal system, it is necessary to take the treatment through at least 3 cycles in order to see the direction of change; however, in this case, after just one period since the initiation of treatment all symptoms were significantly improved, and we were able to proceed with the all-important lifestyle advice to work on the long-term prospects.

THE RESPIRATORY SYSTEM

The respiratory system is the body's way of absorbing oxygen, and it is vital to keep it in good working order. You can survive without food for a couple of weeks; without water for a few days; but without oxygen you'd last only two or three minutes.

Iris signs

The most common signs for respiratory disease are rarefaction and open lacunae within the lung sectors themselves (Figure 9.18), sometimes accompanied by other inflammatory or congestive signs, such as a lymph rosary (this can be partial, affecting on the lung zones), or irritation fibers and transversals. In addition check for kidney signs: rarefaction of both kidney AND lung zones is a well-observed sign in asthmatics (Figure 9.19).

For other affectations of the respiratory tract, such as ear, nose, and throat problems, observe the relevant sectors in the irides, in the context of the overall constitution. For example in a lymphatic type reactivity of the system is assumed and may be evident from early life. In a mixed type problems may be linked to an overproduction of "phlegm" from a poorly functioning digestion. And in a hematogenic constitution any reactivity of the system is automatically regarded as potentially more serious due to the typical delayed symptom development expected in the type.

Herbal choices

People with these signs must focus on immunity, as the implication is that there is an inherited weakness. One of the best herbs to use to support the respiratory tract is astragalus, which comes to us from the Chinese herbal tradition. In my practice, although I do generally prefer to use herbs that grow closer to home, I do use significant amounts of this herb, as it is has many indications, also supporting general immunity, digestion, energy levels and

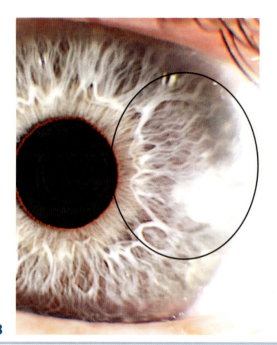

FIGURE 9.18

Large open lacuna/rarefaction in the lung region.

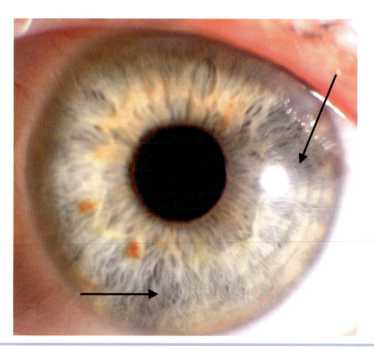

FIGURE 9.19

Rarefaction of both lung and kidney zones.

blood composition. I find it one of the most effective agents in all these situations.

However, if you are suffering with an active pathogen, astragalus is not for you. Infective conditions must be cleared first, before starting with a tonic such as astragalus, and for these purposes echinacea, elecampane, mullein and thyme will be better choices.

For allergic reactivity (hay fever) use nettle, plantain, marshmallow or echinacea. a strong infusion of nettle taken at least three times daily during the hay fever season can work wonders.

For asthma, the following herbs have bronchodilatory effects: elecampane, grindelia (tar weed), licorice, and believe it or not, coffee—as a (recovered) asthmatic of many years I can attest to the benefits of a cup of strong black coffee in managing an asthma attack. It is necessary, however, in addition to treating the acute symptom, to work on the underlying problem—immunity/allergy, overproduction of phlegm and catarrh, the elimination of unhelpful foods such as dairy produce, and stress and anxiety.

General care of the respiratory system

- deep breathing, preferably in fresh, open air;
- exercise, to include aerobic—increases breath rate;
- correcting hunched posture, which compresses lungs;
- keep the digestion active and reduce mucus-forming foods;
- correct response in case of immune challenge (colds, 'flu, etc.)—do not suppress!
- use herbs, natural supplements, homeopathy to address any problems;
- perform regular detoxification routines to clear phlegm and stagnation;
- if you smoke, *stop now*!

THE SKIN

General factors influencing skin disorders include the nervous system (stress and anxiety), disturbed filtration and purification of the blood (liver and kidney function), and the immune system (allergy and autoimmune disturbances).

People who suffer from inflammatory skin problems often notice that their condition worsens under stress. The skin is your boundary with the outer world, and a skin problem may represent a conflict with your environment or close acquaintances. There is sometimes a need to acknowledge irritation, anger, or resentment as part of releasing the condition.

The presence of a *scurf rim* in the iris nearly always signifies involvement of the skin. It may only be dry or itchy skin or it may be eczema or psoriasis. The scurf rim is also a sign for toxicity due to inefficient elimination. This "holding on" also applies to emotions; there may be difficulty admitting to feelings or holding on to difficult feelings.

Iris signs

The iris in Figure 9.20 belongs to a patient who was suffering from chronic eczema. The constitution is lymphatic dyscratic, and the iris has a densely populated fiber structure—a high-resistance type, with sensitivity indicated by the contraction furrows. There is a dark scurf rim. Yellow pigment around the collarette is *hepatotropic*, reflecting possible disturbances with the liver and indicating that allergic tendencies are possibly exacerbated by food choices—dairy produce should be avoided.

Herbal choices

Alterative herbs, or blood purifiers, alongside nervines and relaxants, are effective for conditions such as eczema and psoriasis, working to improve the function of the liver and kidneys. One of my clients, a 49-year-old man, had taken steroids to treat his eczema for so long that his skin was breaking and bleeding every

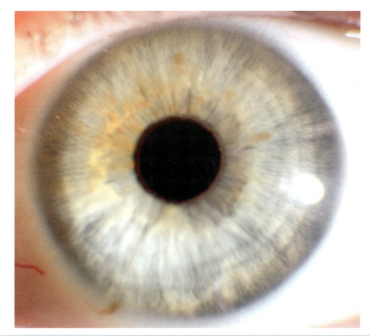

FIGURE 9.20

Iris showing predisposition to eczema, in 48-year-old female.

time he banged it or brushed it. If he stopped the steroids, his eczema flared uncontrollably. We stopped the steroids, cleansed the blood, and balanced the nervous system, and his skin began to regain its stability and structure.

Herbs to consider include red clover flowers, cleavers, burdock root, mountain grape root, alongside nerve relaxing and restorative herbs such as passionflower, skullcap, and oat straw.

THE KIDNEYS AND THE URINARY TRACT

Inadequate kidney function may cause a great many problems, including high blood pressure, skin problems, arthritic and rheumatic disease, asthma, water retention and swelling of the extremities, and other congestive conditions, for example, sinusitis and general lymphatic sluggishness.

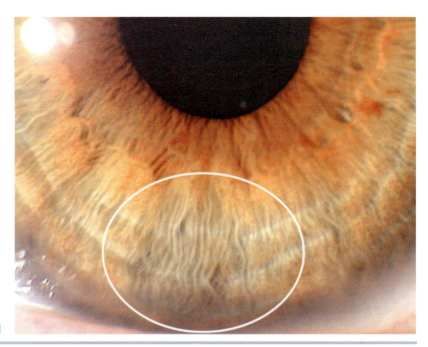

FIGURE 9.21

Rarefaction of fiber structure in the kidney zone; the interruption in contraction furrows in this sector makes it a focus for stress.

You can frequently observe rarefaction, or loosening of the fiber structure, in the kidney zone (see Figure 9.21), an important sign in the assessment of chronic fatigue and debility. There is a close connection between the kidneys and the adrenals. In Chinese medicine, depletion of the kidneys is a noted cause of debility and exhaustion, similar to what Western medicine might refer to as adrenal exhaustion.

The presence of crypts in the kidney zones sometimes shows a tendency to form kidney stones. They also can show that a family member experienced this problem, usually the father. If there is a hyperacidic overlay (cloudy iris), then this tendency is amplified.

Iris signs

The bladder reflex is found in the right iris at 23 minutes and in the left iris at 38 minutes. Whiteness or bright fibers in this sector may reveal a tendency to cystitis or recurrent urinary tract infections. It is also important to look at the smaller reflex sites for the ureters (passages from the kidneys to the bladder) and the urethra (outlet from the bladder).

Treatment

Your water consumption must be adequate; check that you are drinking at least two liters a day.

Herbal choices

Drinking cranberry juice is effective for relieving the symptoms of cystitis. Buchu herb and bearberry, taken as teas or tinctures, act as diuretics and antiseptics; marshmallow root soothes the urinary tract; horsetail and agrimony act as urinary astringents for overfrequent urination and urination at night; and gravel root and hydrangea root are effective for dissolving stones.

A case of kidney stones

Raju is a 40-year-old Nepalese traditional doctor, or medicine man. His symptoms were renal colic (pain as a result of stones trapped in one of the ureters—the narrow tubes leading from kidney to bladder) and hematuria (blood in the urine). The likely cause was kidney stones; however, an ultrasound scan was not conclusive. He had suffered the same problem 18 to 20 years ago.

His life was highly stressful because he was the best-known and most sought-after practitioner in his tradition, and he was also the last surviving person who could preserve this knowledge. He wanted to set up a foundation for the preservation and dissemination of his tradition. He was working extremely hard and had a lot of stress.

His diet was a strong factor in his symptoms. He drank a glass of water and lemon juice every morning, but then drank no water for the rest of the day. At every house call he was offered millet wine, amounting to more than a bottle a day.

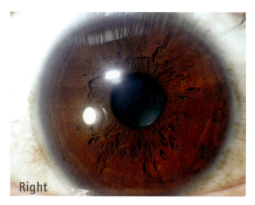
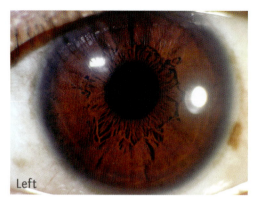

Right   Left

FIGURE 9.22

Raju

His meals were mainly chicken and vegetables with rice, but were always highly salted, and he drank two glasses of cola daily. He was significantly dehydrated and suffered from constipation, passing bowel motions every other day.

Irides

Raju has a pure dark brown hematogenic constitution (Figure 9.22)—irides as dark as these can be difficult to read and need good lighting. There is a tendency toward accumulation of metabolic wastes and a predisposition to toxicity and disorders of blood composition. The formation of stones is fairly common for people of this type.

Loose texture and honeycombs in the nutritive zone suggests a predisposition to constipation and retention of toxins in the gut; however, they also suggest a highly developed instinctual nature and an ability to follow gut feelings.

There is a blue tinge to the edge of the iris, indicating congestion and stagnation of venous circulation, adding to the impression of congestive conditions of the blood. Radial and contraction furrows attest to internalized stress, but also to an ability for focused activity.

There is a honeycomb of deep crypts in the right kidney zone, also frequently associated with kidney insufficiency and the formation of stones.

Treatment

The priority was to dissolve the stones. I helped him to perform a herbal dissolvent routine daily. This involved juicing apples to produce two liters of juice, then bringing this to the boil with an ounce each of gravel root (*Eupatorium purpurea*) and hydrangea root (*Hydrangea arborescens*). Half an ounce of marshmallow root was added to lubricate and soothe the urinary passages. Raju used a sieve when he urinated to see if he passed deposits.

On the second day of this treatment the bleeding had subsided and he passed a 3–4 mm stone with no apparent discomfort. He has not had any repeat of the problem, drinks more water, and eats a less salty diet. Activating the bowels and cleansing the blood formed the second stage of treatment, to help prevent a recurrence.

Passing blood possibly also symbolized a sense of powerlessness and futility, as well as frustration in his mission to protect and preserve his traditional medical knowledge. He eventually succeeded in setting up a foundation for the preservation of this knowledge, and a school in Nepal in which to teach traditional medicine. It was my honor to help in this case, particularly since, having met him through in Cambridge university contacts, he asked for me specifically when he became ill. His associates flew him from Kathmandu to London especially to be treated by me!

NOTES

1. Hauser, W., Karl, J., & Stolz, R. (2000). *Information from Structure and Colour*. Heimsheim: Felke Institut.
2. Christopher, J. R. (1976). *The School of Natural Healing*. Springville, IL: Christopher Publications.
3. Airola, P. (1968). *There Is a Cure for Arthritis*. West Nyack, NY: Parker; reprinted Hoboken, NJ: Prentice Hall, 1988.

10

Natural detoxification and healing protocols

On the following pages, you will find easy detoxification techniques that can be simply and safely performed in your own home yet can be very powerful in both preventive and curative treatments. These routines remove obstructions to health; they detoxify through the eliminative channels of the body and restore healthy functioning to the whole system. They can be used at routine intervals as a preventive measure or as part of a program to restore optimum health after a period of illness.

Your body performs detoxification on a daily basis. However, many of us either exceed "safe" limits of toxic ingestion in our daily diets and through other habits, such as drinking alcohol or smoking, or else we may have inherent tendencies to weaknesses in our eliminative processes. These factors may be aggravated by the effects of physical, emotional, and mental stress.

CASTOR OIL PACKS

Castor oil can be used to break up and draw out congestion through the skin. It can be valuable in relieving symptoms of menstrual disorders and to ease the pain of colitis and diverticulitis. It also can be used to decongest the liver and kidneys. In these cases, packs are applied to the abdomen. Packs also can be applied to the neck, under the arm, or in the groin area to relieve lymphatic swellings.

Conditions to treat

The key word for conditions that may benefit from this treatment is "*congestion.*" Fluids and waste materials build up where the tissues are unable to drain effectively through the usual channels, and this results in congestion.

Congestive disorders

Iridology is very good at picking out areas that may exhibit signs of pain, inflammation, and swellings—the chief symptoms of congestion. If the bowels, kidneys, liver, or the lymphatic vessels are underfunctioning or blocked, they will produce a buildup of waste materials, which then causes inflammation and irritation in the localized area affected.

Pelvic inflammatory disease (PID)

PID is a catch-all disorder for a variety of problems affecting the female reproductive organs, which may include menstrual difficulties, ovarian cysts, fibroids, and endometriosis. Often, abdominal symptoms are found to be a result of constipation or an infrequently evacuated bowel. Fecal matter stored in the sigmoid colon, the "S"-bend at the lower end of the colon, can put pressure, both toxic and mechanical, on the surrounding tissues. The female reproductive organs are in very close proximity, so they suffer the most from any such effect.

Adhesions

An occasional side effect of gynecological or genitourinary surgery, adhesions are another frequent cause of abdominal pain. Even keyhole surgery can have far-reaching consequences in this regard. Whenever you cut the body, it has to repair itself. In order to do this it secretes fibrin, a sort of glue, and in order to make sure the job is done properly, it uses plenty of it. This can result in a "sticking together" of internal tissues and organs, known as adhesions. A castor oil pack is considered a specific remedy for adhesions and will soften, dissolve, and remove the obstruction in a gentle and natural way, yet without "ungluing" the wound itself. You can also use a supplement called serapeptase to help with the internal "digestion" of such material.

To prepare and use a castor oil pack, you will need:

- good quality castor oil: you can buy this in supermarkets, health food shops, or even pharmacies; buy organic where possible;
- a piece of soft, undyed, unbleached cotton cloth;
- some plastic wrap or sheeting;
- a towel;
- a hot water bottle or heat pack.

For problems such as the ones mentioned above, you should follow this routine every other day, or twice a week. Sometimes you may see yellow or brown deposits on the cloth when it is taken off. This indicates that toxins and impurities are being drawn out through the skin. If this happens, the cloth should be thrown away. Otherwise, it can be washed and reused for the next application.

Method:

1. Warm 4–5 tablespoons (50 ml) of castor oil in a pan to a temperature just bearable on the skin.
2. Soak the cloth in the oil for about a minute, then gently squeeze out any excess oil, but do not wring it dry. The cloth should be moist with oil.
3. Position the cloth over the area you are going to treat.
4. Cover the cloth with plastic wrap or sheeting (plastic wrap can be wound around the body to secure the pack in place).
5. Place a towel over the top of the plastic, and a hot-water bottle or hot pack over the towel.
6. Lie down for 30–40 minutes. Shower off when you are finished.

Contraindications

You should not use a castor oil pack if you are pregnant or breast-feeding. Also, you should not apply one to an open wound.

The castor oil plant (*Ricinus communis*) is extremely toxic to humans and animals and can, if ingested, result in death. The toxin contained in castor beans is ricin, a water-soluble protein that is concentrated in the seed, although the rest of the plant is considered to be slightly toxic as well. Commercially prepared castor oil, however, contains no toxins at all.

DRY SKIN BRUSHING

The body eliminates waste products through the skin. To maximize its effectiveness, your skin must be allowed to perform its eliminative function unimpaired. Restrictive artificial fabrics and antiperspirants negatively affect the skin's ability to do so. As well as avoiding these things, we also can stimulate the skin to work more effectively by employing a few simple techniques, including dry skin brushing. This exfoliates the skin and also stimulates the lymph and blood. It leaves you with a pleasant, tingling glow, and over time your skin will attain a satin-like, youthful appearance.

Conditions to treat

Dry skin brushing can be used by anyone, but especially where a scurf rim is seen on the iris, regardless of whether or not there is a skin problem. It is an aid to elimination, reduces the stress on the kidneys, and is part of a general detox program. It improves skin condition, returning lackluster skin to glowing positive health. You can perform skin brushing where there is a skin inflammation, as long as you don't brush over broken or weeping skin.

How to brush your skin

> Use a natural bristle brush (e.g., coconut bristles—these can be bought specifically for the purpose from health food stores). Buy one with a long handle to make brushing your back easier.

> Lightly brush the entire surface of your skin once daily, ideally before showering or bathing. Work in small circles, moving from the extremities in toward the heart.

> Begin with your feet and work up your legs and over your buttocks.

> Then brush your arms, beginning with your hands and working up to your shoulders. Then brush around your rib cage in toward the center and around each breast.

> When you reach your abdomen, brush in a large circle over the abdomen in a clockwise direction following peristaltic flow, around the belly button.

> Finish by softly brushing your face—you can get softer facial brushes for this. Start with the forehead, then work to each side and down past your ears. Brush outward over the cheekbones and down the side of your neck. Do the same over your upper lip and chin, working from the center out, and then down your neck. Finish by brushing down your neck, following the flow of lymphatic drainage.

Contraindications

Do not brush broken skin, acne, or weeping skin conditions such as eczema. Brush around raised moles.

WATER CONSUMPTION

The human body is composed of at least 70% water, and this needs constant cleaning and replacement. You need to drink an average of two liters of pure water a day, but if you drink alcohol, coffee, tea, or carbonated, sugary drinks, you need extra water to compensate for their dehydrating effects. Excess salt in your diet will also increase this need.

If you currently do not drink enough water, try to increase your daily intake over a period of a few weeks by setting yourself targets and increasing the amount slowly. Once you have the habit of drinking more, you will find it easy to maintain, and you will notice the shortfall if you slacken off.

Use the cleanest water it is possible to get. I have tried a number of different solutions to this, and my personal choice is distillation. Distillers can be relatively cheap these days, and I suggest that once tried, you will not look back. Remember, distilled water contains nothing but H_2O: you will see (and smell) on the inside of the distiller kettle whatever else was originally in the water from your tap: it is an education!

However, you can also try filtration of various kinds, with possibly the most complete method being reverse osmosis. This will take out most (but not all) impurities.

HYDROTHERAPY

Water can be used to stimulate circulation and boost the skin's eliminative function, as well as that of the deeper organs of the body. It is a powerful adjunct to any health-building program.

Use hydrotherapy on a daily basis for best results. You can direct water at certain organs or parts of the body that need attention—for example, an aching joint or a congested liver or kidney. Simply by stimulating the circulation in these areas, you will effectively mobilize your body's healing energy in that direction. Saunas and steam baths, with accompanying cold plunges, are included in hydrotherapy. Some spas have hoses that can be used to deliver high-pressure jets of water at specific locations on the body.

Conditions to treat

Hydrotherapy may be used as an integral part of a general detoxification program. However, it may be very successful in the treatment of all kinds of localized problems, from liver congestion to arthritis. It is particularly helpful in cases of chronic inflammation. Arthritic joints benefit not only from the increase in circulation, but also in a reduction in local pain. Water may be directed at specific sites, including the liver, the kidneys, and other internal organs, in order to improve the circulation in those areas.

How to perform
a simple hydrotherapy routine

> After dry skin brushing (see above), get into the shower.

> Direct water, as hot as you can stand, for 30–60 seconds, all over your body.

> Then, with the water as cold as you can take, direct this over your body, for 30–60 seconds.

> Perform this several times, each session lasting for 30–60 seconds. If you start with moderate temperatures, you will find that you can quickly progress to greater extremes of hot and cold.

> Finish by using cold water if you can, though if you suffer from rheumatic or arthritic conditions, it is best to end by using warm water.

Contraindications

Hypermobile joints should not be overheated, and rheumatic joints should not be overchilled. Use warm/cool water if these problems apply. These conditions will improve over time, and tolerance will develop if you persevere.

BOWEL CLEANSES

No detox is complete without attention to the bowel, the body's main exit channel. Cleansing the bowel with herbal remedies, enemas, or colonic hydrotherapy can be an essential part of a healing program. Seek expert advice before considering these routines.

The rationale for bowel cleansing is that the health of the bowel is fundamental to the health of the whole system. Toxins retained in the bowel can leak into the surrounding tissues and the blood, affecting other organs, and may be at the root of many symptoms, such as tiredness, headaches, circulatory difficulties, menstrual and hormonal problems, and immune dysfunction.

The first step to ensuring good bowel health is adequate hydration. Adults need to drink an average of 2 liters of water a day. It is vital that you drink adequate amounts of water if you undertake a bowel cleanse. One of the functions of the colon is to absorb water from the feces. If there is too little water, the feces become dry and sticky, making it more difficult for the body to get rid of them.

It should take about 10–12 hours for material to make the journey through your body. At least one bowel movement for each meal is ideal.

Herbal bowel cleanses operate on a dual principle of cathartic herbs, which stimulate the peristaltic muscles to evacuate, and mucilaginous and demulcent herbs, which soothe the lining of the bowel and provide bulk. In addition to the powders, we add ingredients that absorb any matter adhering to the bowel wall, or in little pockets (diverticuloses) that many of us develop as we grow older.

Conditions to treat

Congestion, systemic toxicity, constipation, liver congestion, menstrual problems, headaches, throat, sinus and immune problems.

Essential ingredients

Seek expert advice on how to perform a bowel cleanse. You can prepare bowel-moving capsules or a formula for absorbing impurities. For bowel-moving capsules, you will need:

> Powders of aloe, cascara, senna, ginger, cayenne, garlic, and barberry root bark. These stimulate peristalsis, correct the gastrointestinal environment, control candida, and boost the body's immunity.

For the formula to absorb impurities, you will need:

> Powders of psyllium husk, linseeds, fennel seeds, slippery elm inner bark, marshmallow root, activated charcoal, bentonite or French green clay, and apple pectin. This absorbs and binds toxic matter and enables efficient elimination.

Contraindications

Consult a professional health practitioner if you have a serious medical condition. The full bowel cleanse may be contraindicated if you have an inflammatory bowel condition such as ulcerative colitis.

ENEMAS

Enemas may be both curative—part of a "get well" program—or preventive. Done on a regular basis, they can strengthen and cleanse the body, increasing its resistance and general stamina. However, they should not be a replacement for natural bowel movements. If you are unable to establish a natural frequency of bowel motions, you should seek help from a herbalist or a colonic therapist.

Enema kits can be obtained for home use; however, it is very important that you get some advice, training, and guidance in how to use them from a trained practitioner.

THE KIDNEY FLUSH OR "MASTER CLEANSER"

This tried and trusted naturopathic routine is simple and effective for detoxifying the kidneys. It can be a regular morning routine, or used on those mornings when you need extra help cleansing and detoxifying your body: for example, if you are feeling sluggish. Mornings are also times when your body is cleansing itself naturally. You will find this routine bracing and stimulating. Do not eat anything before drinking the kidney flush.

Conditions to treat

General congestion, sinusitis, water retention, mild arthritis or rheumatism, poor circulation. As a general occasional mild cleanse.

How to prepare the kidney flush

You will need:

- *2 lemons or 1 lemon and 1 lime, preferably organic and unwaxed*
- *a juicer or blender*
- *half a pint of pure water, cold or hot*
- *cayenne tincture or cayenne powder*
- *maple syrup to sweeten, if desired*

Method

1. Put the lemons and/or lime through the juicer. The skin and pith of citrus fruits contain many beneficial essential oils. Some people experience an occasional tendency to an overacid stomach with these fruits, and the skin and pith counteract this.
2. Add the juice to at least half a pint of pure water. You can use either cold or hot water.
3. Add 10 drops of tincture of cayenne pepper, or a pinch of cayenne powder. If you need to sweeten the drink, add organic maple syrup, not sugar or honey.

Do not eat anything until half an hour after finishing the flush.

Contraindications

If you frequently experience excessive stomach acid and reflux, lemons may exacerbate this. In this case, use half a lemon only, or use apple cider vinegar instead.

THE LIVER FLUSH

This morning routine detoxifies the liver, stimulating it to cleanse itself by dumping bile through the biliary tract into the gastrointestinal tract, making you feel lighter and more energetic. It also is nourishing and supporting to both your immune system and digestion, and will help your body to throw off the threat of viral or bacterial infection.

Perform this routine first thing in the morning before eating. You may feel a little faint or sick at first, or develop a slight headache—this is temporary hypoglycemia (low blood sugar) as a result of not eating when you are used to. If you persevere, this will be cured by the routine. The garlic in the flush is a wonderful remedy for the pancreas, as it works to correct blood sugar imbalances and stimulates the secretion of digestive enzymes.

You should perform the kidney flush for a few days before you start on the liver flush. Then perform the liver flush for ten days consecutively. You can also repeat this flush for one or more days any time you are feeling a bit sluggish, after overindulgence of any kind, or routinely at the change of the seasons, which is a time that tends to put stress on our systems. I advise doing a full liver cleanse every 3 or 4 months.

Conditions to treat

General congestion, digestive bloating and fullness, low immunity, menstrual problems, allergies, skin outbreaks, persistent headaches (check with a medical practitioner first for more serious possibilities).

How to prepare the liver flush

You will need:

- *1 whole lemon, juiced*
- *½ pint organic fresh pressed apple juice*
- *1 tablespoon virgin cold-pressed olive oil*
- *1 clove garlic*
- *small piece fresh ginger root*
- *jug blender*

Method:

1. Juice the lemon in a juicer.
2. Crush, then finely chop the garlic.
3. Grate the ginger.
4. Place all of the ingredients in a blender and liquidize.
5. Pour out and drink slowly.
6. Start preparing the herbal detox tea.

Do not eat anything before drinking the liver flush.

You will also need to prepare a herbal detox tea:

Herbal detox tea

You will need:

- *1 heaped dessertspoon of all or some of following herbs: nettle herb, yellow dock root, dandelion root and leaf, burdock root, red clover flowers, cleavers (these can be used in equal parts).*
- *Add fennel seed, fresh ginger root, fenugreek seed, clove buds, licorice root, orange peel, Pau d'arco bark, juniper berry, black peppercorn, cinnamon bark, cardamom pods in smaller quantities (about ¼ of the amount compared to the herbs in the first list).*
- *2 pints water*

Method

1. Place 1 heaped dessertspoonful of the herb mix in a pan.
2. Add 1 pint of water, bring to the boil, and simmer for 10 minutes with the lid on.
3. Strain the herbs, replace them in the pan with another pint of water, and then repeat.

Drink the first decoction, beginning at least 20 minutes after taking the initial liver flush drink. When the second decoction is ready, carry on drinking. Aim to have at least 2 full mugs of the tea during the 2-hour period of the cleanse.

Do not eat anything for 2 hours after you start this routine, then preferably eat something light; fruit is ideal.

Contraindications

If you have gallstones or a liver disease such as hepatitis, do not use a liver flush without first consulting a professional practitioner.

If you are pregnant, you may do this flush; however, substitute the detox tea with a simple herbal tea: peppermint is ideal.

Contraindications

Avoid the detox tea if you are pregnant or breast feeding; if you suffer from high blood pressure omit the licorice.

HERBAL PREPARATIONS

Infusions, decoctions, tinctures, and teas have a wide range of applications. Throughout the book, for each constitution and problem, certain herbal preparations are recommended. The preparation methods are the same, no matter your iris type, and each has been designed to make the most of the different parts of plants. The herbal detox tea is used in conjunction with the liver flush. It can also be used it for general congestion, water retention, low immunity, and bloating.

Infusion

Use this method for dried leaves, flowers, and "tops" of herbs.

1. Place 2 teaspoonfuls dried herbs in a tea infuser tea-ball.
2. Place the infuser in a cup. Pour freshly boiled water over the herbs.
3. Steep for 10 minutes and then drink the tea.

Alternatively, add 1 dessertspoonful of dried herbs to 1 pint of boiled water in a teapot. Steep, as above, and then drink.

Decoction

Use this method for roots, seeds, barks, and berries.
1. Place 1 dessertspoonful of dried herbs in a saucepan.
2. Add 1 pint of water, bring to a boil, and simmer for 10–15 minutes.
3. Strain and drink.

Tinctures or fluid extracts

Tinctures are alcohol and water extractions, and are very concentrated. They are available from the larger herbal stores and health food shops, and from herbal practitioners. The dose depends on the strength of the extract, but a rough guide is one teaspoon three times a day for tinctures, or half a teaspoon three times a day for fluid extracts.

FOOD COMBINING

Eating and drinking foods in particular combinations can be invaluable for weight loss and for treating certain digestive disorders, as one of its benefits is to facilitate the eliminative functions and maximize digestive power. Well-known versions include the Hay diet, and the "Fit for Life" program.

Conditions to treat

Obesity and weight problems, blood sugar abnormalities, digestive bloating, acid indigestion, and food allergies/sensitivities.

Contraindications

None.

How to combine foods

> Eat fruit only for breakfast. You can eat as much as you like, but try not to eat too many different types at one sitting. In particular, do not combine melons with other fruits. Melon is digested very easily and quickly, even more so than other fruits. If combined with other foods it tends to ferment, causing bloating and discomfort. You may, however, take one or more of the "superfoods" (see below). Your first full meal should be at lunchtime.

> Never eat fruit with any other food type, so don't have it for dessert after a main meal. You need to leave at least half an hour between eating fruit and anything else, and at least two hours after eating a meal before you eat fruit. This is because fruit held up in transit behind heavier foods that take longer to digest will tend to ferment, adding to problems of bloating and dysbiosis.

> Do not drink anything with your meals except a moderate quantity of water, a herbal digestive tea, or vegetable juice. Drinking anything else will dilute digestive secretions and weaken your digestion.

> Eating proteins and carbohydrates together in the same meal used to be contraindicated in food-combining programs. However, this doesn't really work for a vegetarian diet, where proteins and carbohydrates often go together in the same foods. Additionally, a combination of proteins and carbohydrates at each meal can be beneficial to balance blood sugar. The best advice is to eat both these food types in moderation, and in due proportion with the fresh produce— vegetables—that should accompany them. A suitable balance would be ¼ carbohydrates (complex), ¼ protein, ½ fresh vegetables.

> ▸ Never eat after 8 pm. At this time your digestive powers are virtually dormant. Food eaten after this will lie heavily on your stomach and may not, in fact, move far until morning, perhaps contributing to restless and disturbed sleep patterns.
> ▸ Lastly, and most importantly, *never overeat*!

SUPERFOODS

Superfoods is the name given to natural vegetable and plant foods containing above-average nutrition. They may be single foods— alfalfa and other sprouted seeds; spirulina, chlorella, and blue/ green algae—all of which are fresh water algae, and sea vegetables. The latter are particularly rich in minerals. There also are proprietary brands available, combining several sources in one formula, usually in powder form.

Conditions to treat

Fatigue/low energy, immune deficiency, and digestive difficulties (superfoods supply easy energy in cases where digestion struggles to do so). Superfoods also combat the effects of stress and supply extra quantities of nutrients—vitamins, minerals, trace elements, and micronutrients.

Contraindications

Check the ingredients for substances to which you may be allergic, otherwise there are no contraindications.

DEEP BREATHING

As well as helping you feel generally centered and energized, deep breathing is very effective for keeping lymph active. The main lymphatic vessel is the thoracic duct, which passes directly through the diaphragm. As the diaphragm moves with your breath, the thoracic duct is massaged, drawing lymph through your entire system. Most of us breathe shallowly, from our chests, which, apart from preventing us from receiving adequate oxygenation, does not engage the diaphragm.

Deep breathing can be integrated into the busiest lifestyle with some discipline and application. The most important thing is to be comfortable. It can be performed while sitting, lying, or standing. If you are standing, make sure you are standing straight, with your feet hip-width apart; your knees loose, not locked; and your arms relaxed by your sides.

If you wish, as you breathe in, imagine your body filling with white or golden light, penetrating to the deepest parts of yourself. As you breathe out, visualize all the tension, blockages, negativity, toxicity, and congestion flowing out of you.

Sitting

1. Start by relaxing your body. Slowly turn your head to the right, then the left; tilt your chin down, then up.
2. Rotate your shoulders backward and forward a few times.
3. Tilt your pelvis back and forth to release any tensions.
4. Stretch out your legs and flex your ankles back and forth.

Lying down

1. Ensure that your body is aligned symmetrically. Perform a brief check on your limbs and muscles.
2. Starting with your feet and moving upward, relax each part of your body in turn. When you get to your head, also pay attention to your eyes and throat, making sure to consciously release any tension you find in these areas.

Performing deep breathing

1. Begin to breathe in slowly and evenly, drawing your breath deep into your abdomen. Place your hands over your abdomen so that you can feel it rise with your in-breath.
2. Keep breathing in until your breath reaches your upper chest. Do not hold your breath.
3. Release your breath by letting it go naturally, letting gravity take it out with no effort on your part.
4. Repeat this pattern at least ten times on each occasion, and perform the routine as often as you find it helpful. Upon completing the cycle you should feel energized, restored, and enlivened.

STRETCHING

The following exercises allow your body to release tension and also occupy your mind. They can specifically help high-resistance types reduce caffeine and sugar in their diet, if performed habitually at the onset of any cravings they may experience.

How to do stretching exercises

1. Stand. Start by stretching your neck and head, rolling your head from side to side.
2. Bring your shoulders as far up toward your ears as you can, then drop them. Do this several times, then roll your shoulders forward and backward a few times.
3. Clasp your hands in front of you and pull them forward, feeling the stretch across your upper back. Then clasp your hands behind you and pull gently backward, feeling the stretch in your upper chest.
4. Next, bend first to one side, letting your fingers slide down the outside of your thighs as far as you can comfortably go, then the other.

5. Circle your hips a few times, first one way, then the other.
6. Stretch one leg out in front of you, bend your other leg, and bend forward over the stretched leg, feeling the pull on the back of your thigh and calf. Repeat on the other side.
7. Finally, let yourself hang forward, with your knees soft and your arms and hands hanging loose toward your feet. Breathe deeply and relax for a few seconds. When you have finished, be sure to drink a full tumbler of water.

VISUALIZATION

Visualization is used chiefly to reinforce positive messages and improve self-esteem. It also aids meditation, rest, and relaxation.

How to practice visualization

1. Sit, lie down, or stand—whatever is most comfortable for you. Close your eyes and imagine you are in a beautiful location of your choice. This may be somewhere real already known to you, or it may be an imagined location. Make sure to see the detail of the place—what is the landscape like, what colors and textures do you see, what sounds do you hear, what smells do you notice?
2. Make yourself as comfortable as you can in this location. Imagine that everything you could possibly need is readily available to you, that whatever you desire can be manifested immediately. Play with this thought a little, without guilt or judgment. You may fantasize about a delicious meal, for example.
3. When you have satisfied this desire, imagine that you are now free to travel through your own world and create whatever you want in your life. Think of the various different aspects of your life—job, money, relationship, leisure, etc.—and imagine how they would be if they were perfectly aligned with your desires. Go into detail and allow yourself

to fantasize complete fulfilment. Brush aside, just for now, any cynical thoughts that come into your mind telling you that you can never attain this.

4. If there is a particularly difficult problem you are faced with, imagine that it is completely and effortlessly resolved. It doesn't matter what it is—it may be giving up smoking or finding a new job. Whatever it is, focus on the success-ful end result, not the problems of achieving it. Imagine that you have already achieved it.

5. When you have this feeling of success, return again to your ideal location. Look around and take in the environment, before bidding it goodbye, till your next visit, then slowly return to the outside world.

6. Always visualize complete fulfilment, and do not analyze your fantasy. Simply regard it as a positive seed that you have planted, which you are sure will grow into fruition in good time. Wait with certainty and optimism for it to manifest.

*Terms in **bold maroon** type refer to items that may be looked up elsewhere in the Glossary.*

Absorption ring (pupillary ruff): Describes the narrow ring of pigmented tissue at the **inner pupil border**; called the absorption ring, as it is said by some researchers (notably Jensen) to depict the functionality (i.e., absorption capacity) of the inner surface of the gastrointestinal tract.

Acute: An active process having generally a short and relatively severe effect (e.g., fever, inflammation). Opposite of **chronic**.

Anterior border layer [ABL]: The surface layer of the iris, in which **pathochromic signs** may appear, due to the presence of pigment cells that are contained in this layer. The ABL is then also encased in a thin endothelial membrane.

Anterior chamber: The fluid-filled space behind the **cornea**, in front of the **iris**.

ANW: *see* **autonomic nerve wreath**.

Arcus senilis: Also called the "arcus," it consists of a partial ring of whitish plaque in the **cornea**, generally obscuring the outer zone of the iris frontally (sometimes also ventrally), considered to be a deposition of cholesterol, triglycerides, inorganic sodium, and other detritus that may block the arteries. "Senilis" suggests this is usually seen in older people. *See also* **lipemic annulus**.

Autonomic nerve wreath: The ANW, also known as the **border of the collarette (BC)**, the concentric vascular structure which divides the iris disk in two parts, roughly a third of the way into the **stroma** from the **pupillary margin**.

Border of the collarette [BC]: The concentric vascular structure that divides the iris into two parts, roughly two thirds of the way into the stroma from the **pupillary margin**. *See also* **autonomic nerve wreath**.

Central heterochromia: Pigment located over the central portion of the iris only, covering the **pupillary zone (collarette)**, and also perhaps the **humoral zone**. Signifies potential for disturbances of the GI tract.

Cervical: Pertaining to the neck.

Chronic: Long-term pathology, may involve degeneration and nerve damage. Associated with dark signs in the iris. Opposite of **acute**.

Ciliary zone: The outer two thirds (approximately) of the iris disk, between the **collarette** and the **limbus**.

Collarette: Another name for the **pupillary zone**.

Constitution: The makeup and functional habit of the body as determined by the genetic endowment of the individual and modified by environmental and lifestyle factors.

Contraction furrow: Circular groove or furrow in the anterior layers of the iris. Several may appear at once in a concentric pattern. They may circle the iris disk entirely or only partially; they may also be broken in places. They signal the effects of stress upon the system, neuromuscular holding patterns, mineral deficiencies, and metabolic imbalances mediated through the nervous system. Also termed **nerve ring** and **cramp ring**.

Cornea: The transparent membrane that protects the anterior aspect of the eye, partly encapsulating the **anterior chamber**.

Cramp ring: *see* **contraction furrow**.

Crypt: A small dark opening, often rhomboid in shape, in the texture of the iris **stroma**. Almost invariably found at or near—either inside or outside—the **collarette**.

Defect sign: Also known as "defect of substance": a small, black mark, often found inside a **crypt** or **lacuna**. Signifies degenerative process.

Density: A measure of the proximity of iris fibers to each other. Determines **resistance** and recuperative powers.

Depigmentation: Loss of pigment or color in the iris. It has been assumed in some iridology circles that this is a sign of the reestablishment of health: however, in some cases depigmentation may be pathological—i.e., caused by disease or viral or autoimmune disturbance.

Diathesis: Higher-than-average tendency to acquire certain pathologies; regulatory dysfunction, which may be either inherited or acquired.

Disposition: Term referring to **density** and structure of the iris, depicting inherent level and distribution of vitality, **resistance**, and the consequent likely behavior of the individual **constitution**.

Doctrine of signatures: The belief that plants may resemble the body parts they are intended to treat, in terms of color and/or shape

Dyschromia: assumption of metabolic disturbance signified by pigments in the iris. *See* **pathochromic sign**

Epithelium: The exterior or interior (sometimes called "endothelium") lining of any organ.

Flocculations: Light-colored flaky masses usually appearing in the outer zone of the iris.

Heterochromia: Hetero = different; chromia = color.

Honeycomb: A **lacuna** with several "chambers."

Humoral zone: The zone immediately outside the **border of the collarette**. Describes the deep cardiovascular and lymphatic circulation, and has implications for absorption and distribution of nutrients; also hormonal activity.

Hyper-:   Increased.

Hypo-:   Decreased, diminished.

Inner pupil border [IPB]:   the inner edge of the iris.

IPB: *see* **inner pupil border**.

Lacuna: An opening in the iris **stroma**, usually appearing as an oval hole in the texture, although other shapes are frequently seen. Lacunae may be "closed" (completely surrounded or bordered by a fiber structure) or "open" (only partially surrounded or bordered).

Leaf lacuna: A **lacuna** found just outside the **collarette**, with fibers inside resembling the ribs of a leaf. Signifies functional disturbance of the hollow and hormonal organs.

Lesion: A break or breakdown of tissue or texture. In iridology terms, a lesion is usually synonymous with a **lacuna** or **crypt**.

Limbus: The meeting of the outer edge of the iris and the **sclera**.

Lipemic annulus: Opaque whitish ring circling the entire outer zone of the iris; also known (incorrectly) as a cholesterol ring. To be distinguished from the **arcus senilis**.

Lymph rosary: A ring of **tophi** or **flocculations** in the outer iris zone (usually fifth minor zone), found in the hydrogenoid constitution, signifying a tendency toward lymphatic stasis.

Medusa: A type of lacuna usually found in the lung or kidney **reaction fields**, resembling the head of snakes of the mythical Gorgon—a human female with living venomous snakes in place of hair. Also known as a "jellyfish lacuna."

Nasal: Term of orientation: the side of the iris close to the nose.

Nerve ring: *see* **contraction furrow**.

Nutritive zone: also known as the **pupillary zone**, so called as it contains the **reaction field** for the gastrointestinal tract.

Pathochromic sign: A pigment marking in the **anterior border layer** of the iris. To be distinguished from **sectoral heterochromia** or **central heterochromia**. May appear in a variety of colors, from pale yellow to dark brown, color indicating the focus of potential pathology.

Posterior: Situated toward the rear.

Posterior epithelium: The rear-most layer of the iris, facing into the interior eye chamber.

Pupillary margin: Inner edge of the iris bordering the pupil. *See also* **inner pupil border**.

Pupillary ruff: The structure at the inner margin of the pupil, appearing as a red/orange "ruff": it consists of the outermost portion of the **retina** as it curls under the **inner pupil border**. It is an extension of the optic nerve and is the only portion of the nervous system visible to the eye.

Pupillary zone: The circular zone immediately around the pupil; also known as the **collarette** and the **nutritive zone**.

Radial furrow: A radiating crease in the iris tissue, wide at the base and tapered toward the limbus. Major radials start in the **pupillary zone** and cross the **collarette**; minor radials start at the collarette and proceed toward the limbus.

Radii solaris: Another name for **radial furrows**.

Rarefaction: A focal loosening in the fiber structure of the iris **stroma**, indicating lack of resistance in the relevant **reaction field**.

Reaction field: Topographical sector of the iris where organ information is registered.

Reactivity: The ability of the organism to react to threats from toxicity or pathogens: shown by relative shading of the iris stroma or trabeculae.

Resistance: Ability of the organism to resist morbid or threatening influences. Shown by the relative **density** of iris **stroma**.

Retina: The innermost tunic of the eye, an expansion or continuation of the optic nerve, forming the receptor for visual sensation.

Root transversal: A **transversal** with two or more branches.

Schnabel lacuna: *Schnabel* means "beak": sometimes called a "beak lacuna." A lacuna with a sharp point penetrating the **collarette**, signifying a potential tumor. The point of the beak may be rounded (benign) or straight (malignant).

Sclera: The white of the eye: an opaque fibrous membrane that protects the inner eye from injury.

Scurf rim: A darkened outer zone indicating a reflux or reabsorption of toxic material from a poorly eliminating skin. Technically, rarefaction of the outer zone of the iris.

Sectoral heterochromia: Pigmentation of a distinct radial sector of the iris.

Sphincter pupillae: A muscular band in the **nutritive zone/pupillary zone** of the iris, which contracts the pupil.

Spondalarthritic ring: White frosting at the border between the sclera and the iris, usually **nasal**, occasionally **temporal**. Predisposition to arthritis, calcium loss, osteoporosis.

Stroma: The vascular layer constituting the bulk of the iris.

Temporal: Term of orientation: that portion of the iris closest to the temple.

Tophi: see **flocculations**.

Topolabile: Name given to a sign that is significant for its general appearance, rather than its precise topographical position on the iris chart.

Topostabile: Name given to a sign that is important for its precise topographical position on the iris chart.

Trabecula: (plural trabeculae) The vascular fibers that comprise the iris stroma.

Transversal: A trabecular fiber that runs "across the grain."

Vascularization: Loss of the outer sheath of an iris fiber (**trabecula**). The fiber then appears to have a pink thread running through it. A sign of stress or trauma to the organ in the relevant **reaction field**.

Ventral: Term of orientation: the lower portion of the iris.

*Page numbers in **bold maroon** indicate definition of the term.*